BIG®
BOOK
STUDY
GUIDE

THE PREFACE

This book was written by members of Alcoholics Anonymous in Little Rock, Arkansas, following the example of a member in another state.

The only purpose of this book is to enable members of Alcoholics Anonymous to find a new way of living made possible through the study of the Big Book.

We came to the fellowship of Alcoholics Anonymous for many reasons: to get people off our backs, to get out of trouble and to escape the lives we were living.

In the fellowship we acquired a desire to stop drinking. This desire enabled us to exchange a life of drinking and getting into trouble for one of not drinking and going to meetings. Some of us listened to those who said that was all we had to do. Others of us took some of the steps, leaving those we did not like. We found we had grown. Compared to the hellish way we had been living, we thought all our problems were solved. We did not know, however, that we had fallen into the trap of "take some and leave some."

A few of us had taken all the steps and found what we thought was the greatest way of life on earth. We had many years of sobriety, and had given a meaning of this program to many others. But we had ceased to grow.

Our problem was caused by our complacent attitude. God had given us so much, surely we should not expect to go further.

One thing we all agree upon through our weekly study of the Big Book: We have found a new depth and understanding of the program. As we apply this to our lives, we obtain the ultimate promise of the Big Book: "We have found much of heaven and we have been rocketed into a fourth dimension of existence of which we had not even dreamed."

It does not matter why you came, nor does it matter where you are in recovery. Our hope is that you will find in your study group the new way of living that we have found. If you do you will fulfill the purpose of this book.

THE PURPOSE

The purpose of this book is to enable every member of the group to extract as much information as possible from each page of the text book *Alcoholics Anonymous*. This is done through questions and answers, each member being ready for discussion. This leads to a deeper understanding of the text. By helping each member gather information, we enhance his ability to arrive at three conclusions: problem, solution, recovery. Once he has reached this point, he will be following the path of the first 100.

HOW TO BEST USE
YOUR BIG BOOK STUDY GUIDE

The Big Book of Alcoholics Anonymous is the key that can open a new life to the recovering alcoholic who is willing to change. This Study Guide will help you achieve a better understanding of the Big Book.

By following the formula of study contained in this Guide Book, you will learn to unlock the power contained within the pages of the Big Book. Here is how it works.

1. Open your Big Book to the Preface, Page XI. Read this page. (Because the Big Book is a textbook, the information is presented in a logical sequence. We recommend that you begin at the beginning, rather than pick and choose pages at random, so that you may gain the most from your Big Book studies.)

2. Turn in the Study Guide to the page number that matches the page you have just read in the Big Book, Page XI. (Page numbers in your Guide Book match the page numbers in the Third Edition of the Big Book.)

3. Answer each question in the Study Guide, referring to the Big Book for the correct answer.

   NOTE: The transparent plastic line guide will help you answer the questions. Here's an example of how to use the line guide. You have already opened your Big Book to Page XI, the Preface. Align the plastic line guide so that 1 _____ is immediately below the top line of type on the page, which reads: "This is the third edition of the book, 'Alcoholics'." Now look at the first question in the Study Guide for Page XI: "1. What has the book become? PXI L7-8." Check the line guide for the correct answer on lines 7-8: "...this book has become the basic text for our society..."

4. After you answer the questions, use a highlighter marker or a pencil to underline words and phrases in the Big Book that you want to recall or study at a later time.

5. Write notes in the margins of your Big Book pages so that you can refer to them in the future.

IT'S THAT EASY! And studying this way will help you achieve a working knowledge and a deeper understanding of the textbook for your recovery. By following this simple formula, you will not only help yourself, but you will be able to help other alcoholics when you progress to Twelfth Step work.

GROUP GUIDELINES

Group members can discuss each question to any length needed as long as they stick to that question only.

1. Each group member should read a paragraph of the material to be discussed.
2. The first person selected at a starting point by the group leader should read the first question and find the answer. He should then make his comment if he has one and ask the members of the group for their comments on this question.
3. The group leader should ask the next group member to read the next question and do the same.

This Big Book discussion meeting must not be confused with an open discussion meeting. The subject to be discussed must be controlled by the question so that the group can concentrate on the text.

Special Note: Most full pages of the Big Book have 33 lines. Because of irregular spacing, some contain fewer and others have more. In such cases, the line-finding sheet will not follow the lines exactly and will have to be moved a little to find the correct lines and answers. When this happens, a note at the bottom of the page will tell the number of lines on such pages.

PREFACE

1. What has the book become?
   P XI   L 7-8

2. Why has it not been changed?
   P XI   L 9-10

3. Has the doctor's opinion been changed?
   P XI   L 14-17

4. What has been added to the first book?
   P XI   L 18-20

5. Why was the history section changed?
   P XI   L 20-22

6. What is the nickname for this volume?
   P XII   L 6-7

FOREWORD TO FIRST EDITION

1. How many helped write this book?
   P XIII   L 1-4

2. What is the main purpose of this book?
   P XIII   L 4-5

3. Is the alcoholic a sick person?
   P XIII   L 9-10

4. Is this book for alcoholics only?
   P XIII   L 11-12

5. Why did the first 100 remain anonymous?
   P XIII   L 13-19

6. How should an AA member identify himself when speaking publicly?
   P XIII   L 20-23

7. What does AA ask of the press?
   P XIII   L 24-26

8. Is AA an organization?
   P XIII   L 27   P XIV   L 1

FOREWORD TO FIRST EDITION

1. How much does it cost to become a member of AA?
   P XIV   L 1-2

2. What is the only requirement to become a member?
   P XIV   L 2-3

3. Is AA allied with other groups?
   P XIV   L 3-5

4. Whom does AA wish to help?
   P XIV   L 5-6

FOREWORD TO SECOND EDITION

1. What has happened since this book was written?
   P XV   L 1-3

2. How many years elapsed between the two editions?
   P XV   L 8-10

3. Where were the groups formed?
   P XV   L 13-22

4. Where did AA start?
   P XV   L 23-24

5. What year did AA start?
   P XV   L 24

6. How did it get started?
   P XV   L 24-26

7. What relieved the broker's obsession?
   P XV   L 26   P XVI   L 1

FOREWORD

1. Who else did the broker meet?
   P XVI   L 1-2

2. Whom had this friend been in contact with?
   P XVI   L 2-3

3. Who helped the broker?
   P XVI   L 3-4

4. What has Doctor Silkworth become?
   P XVI   L 5-6

5. What did the broker learn from the doctor?
   P XVI   L 8-9

6. Could he completely accept all the program of the Oxford Group?
   P XVI   L 9-10

7. What parts of the Oxford Group did he use?
   P XVI   L 10-14

8. Before going to Akron, what had Bill been doing?
   P XVI   L 15-17

9. Whom did he help?
   P XVI   L 17-18

10. What did he go to Akron for?
    P XVI   L 18-19

11. What was he afraid of?
    P XVI   L 20-21

12. What did he do to save himself?
    P XVI   L 21-23

FOREWORD

13. To whom did he carry the message?

    P XVI   L 23-24

14. How had the physician tried to resolve the alcoholic dilemma?

    P XVI   L 25-26

15. Had he been successful?

    P XVI   L 26

16. What did the broker give the physician?

    P XVI   L 26-28

17. With this new information, did the physician succeed?

    P XVI   L 28-32

18. What did this seem to prove?

    P XVI   L 32   P XVII   L 1

FOREWORD

1. What else does this experience indicate?
   P XVII   L 1-3

2. Where did the two men start their work?
   P XVII   L 4-6

3. Were they successful?
   P XVII   L 6-8

4. When was the first AA group formed?
   P XVII   L 8-13

5. As the membership grew, what were they convinced of?
   P XVII   L 14-17

6. Where were the AA groups in 1937?
   P XVII   L 18-22

7. What did these struggling groups do?
   P XVII   L 23-25

8. What did these efforts produce?
   P XVII   L 25-26

9. How many members were in these groups when the book was published?
   P XVII   L 26-27

10. Where did AA get its name?
    P XVII   L 28-30

FOREWORD

1. What was the first magazine article written about AA?
   P XVIII   L 1-4

2. What did the article do for the AA movement?
   P XVII   L 4-7

3. In what other way was the AA message carried?
   P XVIII   L 9-14

4. Who else helped AA get moving in the early days?
   P XVIII   L 15-20

5. What was the second magazine to produce a feature article on AA?
   P XVIII   L 21-27

6. What was the next great question to face a growing AA?
   P XVIII   L 29   P XIX   L 2

FOREWORD

1. Did these problems come about in AA?
   P XIX   L 2-3

2. What was AA's conviction?
   P XIX   L 3-6

3. Without unity, what would have happened?
   P XIX   L 6-7

4. What were the next principles developed?
   P XIX   L 8-24

5. When were the traditions accepted by the fellowship?
   P XIX   L 25-30

6. What is one of AA's assets?
   P XIX   L 30-31

FOREWORD

1. Why did the public accept AA?

   P XX   L 1-5

2. What was the recovery rate of AA in the early days?

   P XX   L 5-12

3. What other field of endeavor accepted AA?

   P XX   L 13-20

4. Is AA a religious organization?

   P XX   L 21-22

5. Does AA have any medical viewpoint?

   P XX   L 22-24

6. What makes everyone even in AA?

   P XX   L 25-28

7. What religions are represented in AA?

   P XX   L 28-30

8. What percentage are women?

   P XX   L 30-31

9. By what rate is AA increasing a year?

   P XX   L 32-33

FOREWORD

1. Will AA help every alcoholic?
   P XXI   L 2-5

2. Is there other therapy for the alcoholic?
   P XXI   L 5-6

3. What do we hope for those who have not found an answer?
   P XXI   L 6-9

FOREWORD TO THIRD EDITION

1. When did the third edition go to the printer?

   P XXII   L 1-2

2. How many were in our fellowship?

   P XXII   L 2-5

3. What percentage were women?

   P XXII   L 9

4. What percentage of new members are women?

   P XXII   L 10-11

5. What is the average age of the new members?

   P XXII   L 11-13

6. Do the 12 steps work all over the world?

   P XXII   L 14-22

7. Although AA has grown, what simple sharing is the core to its success?

   P XXII   L 23-27

THE DOCTOR'S OPINION

1. Why did AA ask Doctor Silkworth to write the Doctor's Opinion for the Big Book?

   P XXIII   L 1-6

2. What was Doctor Silkworth's position and where was he working?

   P XXIII   L 7-9

3. In what field had the doctor become a treatment specialist?

   P XXIII   L 11-12

4. How did Doctor Silkworth consider Bill's condition when he came to the Towns Hospital in late 1934?

   P XXIII   L 13-16

5. How many times was Bill treated at the Towns Hospital?

   P XXIII   L 17-18

28 lines on this page

THE DOCTOR'S OPINION

1. In 1934 with only 100 people sober, what did Doctor Silkworth believe the AA program could become?

   P XXIV L 2-3

2. Did he have faith in 100 drunks?

   P XXIV L 4-5

3. What two parts of human life are affected by the disease of alcoholism?

   P XXIV L 8-13

4. Does this illness affect the mind?

   P XXIV L 10-16

5. Is the body of the alcoholic sick?

   P XXIV L 18-21

6. Can we completely understand alcoholism if we leave out the physical factor?

   P XXIV L 18-19

7. Was the doctor's idea based on fact?

   P XXIV L 22-23

8. What did the first 100 think of this theory?

   P XXIV L 23-24

9. As laymen in the field of medicine, could they prove or disprove this theory?

   P XXIV L 23-24

10. What did it explain to the ex-problem drinker?

    P XXIV L 26-27

11. The problem is physical and mental. Where is the solution?

    P XXIV L 28-29

12. Why did the doctor favor hospitalization?

    P XXIV L 29-30

13. When the brain is cleared, what condition improves?

    P XXIV L 2 P XXV L 2

THE DOCTOR'S OPINION

1. How important is the subject in this book to those who suffer from alcoholism?

   P XXV   L 4-6

2. What was the doctor's experience in this field?

   P XXV   L 7-9

3. Was Doctor Silkworth proud to be a part of the AA effort?

   P XXV   L 10-12

4. How does the AA book cover the subject of alcoholism treatment?

   P XXV   L 11-12

5. What had the doctor realized for a long time?

   P XXV   L 13-14

6. Though doctors knew that something drove the alcoholic to self-destruction, why had they not been able to identify and understand this fact?

   P XXV   L 16-19

7. What did Bill do with the idea he acquired?

   P XXV   L 20-23

8. After his recovery using these ideas, which step did he work?

   P XXV   L 22-23

9. How did the doctor feel about Bill talking to his other patients?

   P XXV   L 24-26

10. What were the results?

    P XXV   L 26-27

11. Was this work done for profit?

    P XXV   L 28-31

THE DOCTOR'S OPINION

12. Was this work inspiring to the doctor?

   P XXV   L 28-31

13. What two things does the recovered alcoholic believe in?

   P XXV   L 31-33

14. Where were the chronic alcoholics pulled back from?

   P XXV   L 33

15. Is the craving caused by the body or the mind?

   P XXV   L 34   P XXVI   L 1

34 lines on this page

THE DOCTOR'S OPINION

1. What is the manifestation of the allergy?
   P XXVI L 4-6

2. Does the average temperate drinker crave alcohol when he drinks?
   P XXVI L 7-8

3. Can alcoholics ever safely use alcohol?
   P XXVI L 8-9

4. What kind of message will interest and hold the alcoholic?
   P XXVI L 14-16

5. What must happen if we are to recreate our lives?
   P XXVI L 16-18

6. Why do men and women drink?
   P XXVI L 30-31

7. Why can't the alcoholic differentiate the true from the false?
   P XXVI L 31-33

8. What is the state of the alcoholic's mind preceding the first drink?
   P XXVI L 34-35

9. What is their relief from this state of mind?
   P XXVI L 35 P XXVII L 3

35 lines on this page

XXVII

THE DOCTOR'S OPINION

1. After they take a drink, what develops?

   P XXVII   L 3-4

2. What does the craving cause?

   P XXVII   L 5-6

3. How can the alcoholic recover?

   P XXVII   L 7-9

4. What does the psychic change enable the alcoholic to do?

   P XXVII   L 10-14

5. What effort is necessary?

   P XXVII   L 15-16

6. Can the doctor produce this psychic change?

   P XXVII   L 17-24

7. Has psychiatric effort been able to help many alcoholics?

   P XXVII   L 24-27

8. Do all alcoholics respond to psychological approaches?

   P XXVII   L 27-28

9. Is alcoholism a problem of mental control?

   P XXVII   L 29-30

10. What did the men do in order to complete their business deal?

    P XXVII   L 30-33

11. What did they do before the deal was completed?

    P XXVII   L 31-32

12. What happens when they take a drink?

    P XXVII   L 32-33

13. What became more important than their business?

    P XXVII   L 33

14. Did they take care of their business?

    P XXVII   L 33   P XXVIII   L 1

35 lines on this page

THE DOCTOR'S OPINION

1. Were these men drinking to escape?
   P XXVIII   L 1-2

2. Is the physical craving stronger than the mental control?
   P XXVIII   L 2-3

3. What does the craving cause men to do?
   P XXVIII   L 4-6

4. What are the five classifications of alcoholics described by Doctor Silkworth?
   P XXVIII   L 8-23

5. What do all classes of alcoholics have in common?
   P XXVIII   L 24-29

6. What is the only relief from the allergy?
   P XXVIII   L 30-31

35 lines on this page

THE DOCTOR'S OPINION

The doctor gives the solution to alcoholism by discussing the cases of two chronic alcoholics who have recovered.

Case 1—P XXIX   L 3-20

Case 2—P XXIX   L 21   P XXX   L 1-end

Can anyone in the group find the solution to the problem found in both cases?

WORD DEFINITIONS
THE DOCTOR'S OPINION

PAGE XXIII

CONCEPTION: a general idea or understanding

FELLOWSHIP: a group of people with the same interests or experiences

PAGE XXIV

INHERENT: existing in someone or something as a natural and inseparable quality

EPOCH: an event or a time that begins a new period or development

ANNALS: history

ABNORMAL: not natural

MALADJUSTED: lacking harmony with one's environment

REALITY: the truth

MENTAL: relating to the mind (mind power)

DEFECTIVE: lacking something essential to be complete

SICKENED: causing sickness

THEORY: a plausible principle used to explain something

ALLERGY: an abnormal reaction to a food or chemical substance

LAYMEN: people who do not have special or advanced training or skills

OPINION: a belief or conclusion held with confidence but not substantiated by positive knowledge or proof

SOUNDNESS: correctness

ALTRUISTIC: concern for the welfare of others as opposed to egoism or selfishness

JITTERY: nervous, uneasy

BEFOGGED: confused

IMPERATIVE: mandatory

PARAMOUNT: of chief concern or importance; primary; foremost

DRUG: a substance other than food taken into the body that changes its function

ADDICTION: state of being given up to some habit, practice or pursuit

ALCOHOL: C_2H_6O (ethyl alcohol)

MORAL: concerned with the principles of right and wrong behavior

PSYCHOLOGY: the science of mind and behavior

ULTRA-MODERN: the very latest

SCIENTIFIC: relating or exhibiting the methods or principles of science

SYNTHETIC: produced artificially; manmade

MISGIVING: a feeling of doubt or suspicion concerning a future event

CONSENTED: to give approval of what is asked

CHRONIC: constantly present; frequently recurring

CRAVING: an abnormal desire; a great desire or longing

PSYCHOLOGICAL: pertaining to psychology (mind and behavior)

MANIFESTATION: something easily perceived by the senses or mind

PHENOMENON: something known by the senses but not understood by the mind

TEMPERATE: exercising moderation and self-restraint

CYNICAL: distrustful of human nature; inclined to question the sincerity and goodness of people

DIFFERENTIATE: recognize a difference

ELUSIVE: evasive; hard to comprehend or define

IMPUNITY: without punishment, harm or loss

SUCCUMBED: yielded to superior strength or force

SPREE: a drinking bout

PSYCHIC: pertaining to the mind

INADEQUACY: insufficiency

AGGREGATE: the sum total

PSYCHOPATH: a person with a personality disorder, especially one manifested in aggressively antisocial behavior

EMOTIONALLY: related to feelings

UNSTABLE: tending strongly to change; not constant; fluctuating

REMORSEFUL: feeling guilt for past wrongs

RESOLUTION: a strong vow or promise

MANIC-DEPRESSIVE: having a mental disorder marked by excitation and depression

SYMPTOM: evidence of disease

DISTINCT: distinguished as not being the same; not identical

ENTITY: something that exists on its own

PERMANENTLY: fixed and changeless

ERADICATED: done away with completely

ABSTINENCE: willful avoidance of pleasure, especially of food and drink

PRECIPITATES: causes to happen

SCOPE: the range of one's perception, thought or action

PSYCHIATRIC: the medical study, diagnosis, treatment and prevention of mental illness

GASTRIC HEMORRHAGE: bleeding pertaining to the stomach

PATHOLOGICAL: pertaining to disease

DETERIORATION: becoming worse

DIAGNOSIS: identifying a disease

IMPULSE: a sudden urge

WILL POWER: strong determination

SPECIMEN: an individual item or part representative of a class or whole

SCOFF: to show or treat with contempt by derisive acts or language

CHAPTER 1
BILL'S STORY

1. Where did Bill discover liquor?

   P 1   L 7

2. When did Bill begin to "use" alcohol?

   P 1   L 10

3. When did his imagination become unrealistic?

   P 1   L 22-26

BILL'S STORY

1. When was Bill's first employment?

   P 2   L 1-2

2. When did he begin to display grandiose thinking?

   P 2   L 2-6

3. When did Bill's drinking begin to cause him problems?

   P 2   L 7-10

4. When did Bill's drinking begin to cause problems in the home.

   P 2   L 10-11

5. When did Bill begin to rationalize his behavior?

   P 2   L 11-15

6. How did Bill choose his stockbroker profession?

   P 2   L 16-22

BILL'S STORY

1. How does Bill describe his early success?
   P 3   L 13-14

2. What part did drinking play?
   P 3   L 17-18

3. What proportion did his drinking assume?
   P 3   L 22-23

4. How did this affect his friendships?
   P 3   L 23-25

5. How was his home life affected?
   P 3   L 25-26

6. How was Bill beginning to feel in the morning?
   P 3   L 32-end

BILL'S STORY

1. How did Bill react to calamity and failure?

   P 4   L 13-16

2. What happened as he drank?

   P 4   L 18-19

3. What happened with his generous Canadian friend?

   . P 4   L 24-26

4. What did they do then?

   P 4   L 27

5. What did his wife do?

   P 4   L 31-end

32 lines on this page

BILL'S STORY

1. How had his career changed?

   P 5   L 1-2

2. What had liquor become?

   P 5   L 3

3. When did Bill begin morning drinking?

   P 5   L 7-11

4. What did Bill think about his condition?

   P 5   L 11-13

5. What happened to Bill's "promising business opportunity"?

   P 5   L 17-21

6. Where did Bill first try to stop drinking on will power?

   P 5   L 22-26

7. How well did his will power work?

   P 5   L 27-29

8. What did Bill begin to wonder?

   P 5   L 31-32

9. As time passed, what was his confidence replaced by?

   P 5   L 33   P 6   L 2

BILL'S STORY

1. Did Bill become overconfident?
   P 6   L 2-3

2. What happened to Bill?
   P 6   L 4-5

3. What did he decide to do after he started to drink?
   P 6   L 5-7

4. Did Bill have hangovers?
   P 6   L 8-10

5. Did Bill have an abnormal fear?
   P 6   L 10-11

6. How did Bill treat his fears?
   P 6   L 14-15

7. How long did Bill endure this agony?
   P 6   L 22-23

8. How did he sometimes finance his morning drinking?
   P 6   L 23-25

9. What did he again think about doing?
   P 6   L 25-27

10. How did he and his wife seek escape?
    P 6   L 28-29

11. Did Bill think about suicide?
    P 6   L 29-32

12. Did Bill have medical help?
    P 6   L 33   P 7   L 1

BILL'S STORY

1. What was Bill's physical condition at this point?
   P 7   L 4-5

2. Where was Bill placed then?
   P 7   L 7-9

3. Whom did Bill meet and what was he told?
   P 7   L 11-13

4. What did Bill learn?
   P 7   L 14-17

5. How did Bill fare with his new understanding of himself?
   P 7   L 18-22

6. What happened once more?
   P 7   L 23-24

7. Did Bill return to treatment?
   P 7   L 25-26

8. What was his wife informed of?
   P 7   L 27-31

9. How did this information affect Bill?
   P 7   L 33   P 8   L 7

BILL'S STORY

1. Where did Bill take step 1?

   P 8   L 8-12

2. Did fear sober him a bit?

   P 8   L 14

3. What happened again?

   P 8   L 14-16

4. What did everyone believe about him at this point?

   P 8   L 16-18

5. After Bill reached his bottom, what was to be the outcome?

   P 8   L 19-24

6. How long had Bill been drinking when Ebby came to see him?

   P 8   L 15-25

7. Did Bill hide his gin?

   P 8   L 26-31

8. Who called Bill and what was the caller's condition?

   P 8   L 32   P 9   L 1

BILL'S STORY

1. What was Bill's reaction to Ebby?
   P 9   L 3

2. What was Bill looking forward to?
   P 9   L 5-8

3. How does Bill describe his friend's coming to visit?
   P 9   L 9-11

4. What was his appearance?
   P 9   L 12-14

5. What did Bill offer?
   P 9   L 15

6. What did Bill's friend tell him?
   P 9   L 19-20

7. What did Bill suspect about him?
   P 9   L 21-22

8. What did he relate to Bill?
   P 9   L 27-32

9. We know Bill has gotten step 1 from Dr. Silkworth, but how does he get the other steps?
   P 9   L 29-31

10. Why had he come to see Bill?
    P 9   L 33   P 10   L 1

BILL'S STORY

1. How did Bill react?

   P 10   L 1-2

2. Why was Bill interested?

   P 10   L 2

3. Who and what influenced Bill's early religious attitudes?

   P 10   L 4-13

4. Was Bill an atheist?

   P 10   L 16-18

5. What does an atheist believe?

   P 10   L 18-20

6. What do the scientists believe?

   P 10   L 20-24

7. How far did his beliefs go?

   P 10   L 26-28

8. Why couldn't he believe in a personal God?

   P 10   L 30-end

BILL'S STORY

1. What did Bill think about Christ's teachings?
   P 11   L 1-5

2. What was Bill's opinion of church people?
   P 11   L 2

3. Where did Bill get his idea about religion?
   P 11   L 6-13

4. But what did his friend declare?
   P 11   L 14-16

5. Which step had Bill and Ebby accepted at this point?
   P 11   L 16-19

6. Where had this power originated?
   P 11   L 22-24

7. What did Bill think about miracles after this?
   P 11   L 26-29

32 lines on this page

BILL'S STORY

1. After all this proof, was Bill still prejudiced about God?

   P 12   L 3-12

2. What did his friend suggest to end this ridiculous argument about religion?

   P 12   L 13-15

3. What effect did this have on Bill?

   P 12   L 16-18

4. Where did Bill take step 2?

   P 12   L 19-23

5. What did coming to believe do to Bill?

   P 12   L 25-28

BILL'S STORY

1. Why did Bill go back to the hospital for the third time?
   P 13   L 3-5

2. Where did Bill take step 3?
   P 13   L 6-10

3. Where did he take step 4?
   P 13   L 10-11

4. Where did he take steps 6 and 7?
   P 13   L 11-12

5. Where did he take step 5?
   P 13   L 14-15

6. Where did he take step 8?
   P 13   L 15-18

7. Where did he take step 9?
   P 13   L 18-20

8. Where did Bill take step 10?
   P 13   L 21-23

9. Where did Bill take step 11?
   P 13   L 21-28

10. What did his friend promise would happen as a result of these steps?
    P 13   L 29   P 14   L 2

11. What step is this? Group Answer

BILL'S STORY

1. Is the AA program complicated?

   P 14 L 3

2. Is the AA program easy?

   P 14 L 3

3. What price do we have to pay for recovering?

   P 14 L 3-4

4. Is alcohol the only thing we turn over to God?

   P 14 L 4-6

5. What kinds of proposals are these?

   P 14 L 7

6. Did Bill have a spiritual experience or a spiritual awakening?

   P 14 L 8-14

7. In what two ways does God come to men?

   P 14 L 13-14

8. What did Bill do when this experience occurred?

   P 14 L 15-16

9. What did he ask the doctor?

   P 14 L 16

10. What was the doctor's answer?

    P 14 L 18-21

11. When and where did Bill conceive the idea that became AA?

    P 14 L 23-27

12. What did Ebby emphasize to Bill?

    P 14 L 28-32

13. How do alcoholics enlarge their spiritual lives?

    P 14 L 33 P 15 L 1

BILL'S STORY

1. What happens to alcoholics who do not work with others to grow spiritually?

   P 15   L 2-5

2. What did Bill and his wife give up everything to do?

   P 15   L 6-8

3. Was Bill able to work?

   P 15   L 8-10

4. Was Bill well? What trouble did he seem to have in his early years of sobriety?

   P 15   L 10-12

5. Did Bill come close to drinking?

   P 15   L 12-13

6. What kept Bill from drinking?

   P 15   L 13-18

7. What did Bill see as a healing miracle that took place?

   P 15   L 19-29

8. Did the program ever fail?

   P 15   L 29-31

9. Where were the largest AA meetings in the early days of AA?

   P 15   L 31   P 16   L 1

BILL'S STORY

1. How many people were at these meetings when this book was written?

   P 16   L 1-2

2. Are drunks sometimes funny?

   P 16   L 4-6

3. Are they tragic?

   P 16   L 4-6

4. Why did Bill's friend commit suicide, and where did this happen?

   P 16   L 6-7

5. Is there fun in the recovery?

   P 16   L 9-11

6. But what else is also there?

   P 16   L 11-12

7. How long does faith have to work?

   P 16   L 12-13

8. What will happen if faith does not work?

   P 16   L 13

9. Have some of us found heaven?

   P 16   L 14-15

10. What has happened to Ebby's message? Where has it gone and what has it become?

    P 16   L 15-18

WORD DEFINITION
BILL'S STORY

PAGE 1
PLATTSBURG: New England town

SUBLIME: lofty, grand, splendid

HILARIOUS: cheerful, boisterous, funny

DOGGEREL: verse that is loosely styled and irregular in measure, used especially for burlesque or comic effect

OMINOUS: foretelling evil; threatening

PAGE 2
MAELSTROM: turbulence

FOREBODINGS: a dark sense of impending evil; an evil omen

PHILOSOPHIC: characterizing a philosopher; enlightened; wise; thoughtful

ALLOY: mixture

SIDECAR: a one-wheeled car for a single passenger, attached to the side of a motorcycle

PAGE 3
LUNACY: unsoundness of mind; insanity; great foolishness; extreme folly

SPECULATION: assuming a business risk in hope of gain

PROCURED: got possession of; obtained; brought about; achieved

EXHILARATING: cheerful or jolly; filled with a lively sense of well-being

REMONSTRANCES: speeches or gestures of protest, opposition or reproof

TERMINATED: brought to an end or halt; concluded; finished

SUMPTUOUS: expensive, luxurious

INFIDELITY: marital unfaithfulness

SCRAPES: quarrels

WALTER HAGEN: professional golfer of the 1920s

JITTERY: nervous, uneasy

PAGE 4

CAROM: collide with a rebound; glance

IMPECCABLE: without flaw; faultless

SKEPTICISM: a doubting or questioning attitude or state of mind; disbelief

ABRUPTLY: unexpectedly, suddenly

PAGE 5

"BATHTUB" GIN: homemade alcohol

PRODIGIOUS BENDER: enormous drinking; spree

PERSPECTIVE: the power to see or think of things in their true relationship to each other

RESOLVE: determination

PAGE 6

COCKSURENESS: overconfidence

GIN MILLS: drinking establishments; bars

CALAMITY: a major misfortune or loss; disaster

WRITHING: twisting and turning this way and that (writhe in pain)

SLENDER: limited or inadequate in amount; meager

PAGE 7

SEDATIVE: a drug that calms or eases tension

MY BROTHER-IN-LAW: a physician, Dr. Leonard Strong

NATIONALLY KNOWN HOSPITAL: Towns Hospital

BELLA-DONNA TREATMENT: a sedative (no longer in use) used on the digestive tract, often in cases of nausea or diarrhea

HYDROTHERAPY: the use of water in the treatment of disease

GOOSE BEING HIGH: a period of good times

DELIRIUM: a mental disturbance characterized by confusion, disordered speech and hallucinations

WET BRAIN: brain damage caused by drinking

ASYLUM: an institution for the care of the mentally ill

DEVASTATING: brought to ruin; overwhelming

PAGE 8
PRIDE: self-respect

SURMOUNT: surpass or exceed in amount; overcome; conquer

OBSTACLE: something that stands in the way of progress toward some goal

SOTS: chronic drunkards

MORASS: something that traps or impedes

SELF-PITY: dwelling on one's sorrows or misfortunes

QUICKSAND: a bed of loose sand mixed with water forming a soft, shifting mass that yields easily to pressure and tends to suck down any object resting on its surface

OVERWHELMED: crushed, submerged

INSIDIOUS: harmful but enticing; treacherous; seductive

INSANITY: not whole of mind

DEBAUCH: extreme imtemperance

CATAPULTED: launched, thrown

MUSING: thinking; contemplation

PAGE 9
RUMOR: unverified information of uncertain origin, usually spread by word of mouth; gossip; hearsay

JAG: a bout or spree

OASIS: a small place preserved from surrounding unpleasantness

RANTING: violent, loud, vehement

SIMPLE RELIGIOUS IDEA: step 2

PRACTICAL PROGRAM OF ACTION: recovery steps 3 through 12

PAGE 10
PROFFERED: suggested

TEMPERANCE PLEDGE: a promise to obstain from drinking

COMTEMPT: disdain; bitter scorn; often disrespect or willful disobedience of authority

IMMUTABLE: not subject to change or alteration

PAGE 11
FACILITATED: made easier

NEGLIGIBLE: so small so as not to merit attention; trifling

POINT-BLANK: clearly, directly

SCRAP HEAP: left over and unwanted; worthless; junk in a pile

MIRACLE: divine intervention in human affairs

TIDINGS: information; news (tidings of great joy)

PAGE 12
VESTIGES: visible traces; evidence or signs of something that has once existed but exists or appears no more

ANTIPATHY: a strong feeling of aversion or opposition

INTENSIFIED: strengthened, sharpened

CONCEPTION: a general idea or understanding

INTELLECTUAL: rational rather than emotional

BELIEVE: accept as true or real

PAGE 13
DEFICIENCIES: defects, inadequacies

RESENTMENT: ill will felt because of a real or imagined offense

WRONG: harm done others

PAGE 14
REVOLUTIONARY: radical, extreme

DRASTIC: especially severe; extreme

THE DOCTOR: Doctor Silkworth

IMPERATIVE: mandatory

CHAPTER 2
THERE IS A SOLUTION

1. Have others found the same answer that Bill found?

   P 17   L 1-3

2. What kind of people make up the fellowship of AA?

   P 17   L 5-8

3. What is their livelihood?

   P 17   L 6

4. What is their religion?

   P 17   L 7-8

5. Should they have even met?

   P 17   L 8-9

6. What exists between them?

   P 17   L 9-11

7. Why are they so close?

   P 17   L 11-14

8. What binds them?

   P 17   L 17-20

9. What warning does this book give?

   P 17   L 19-20

10. What else do these people have in common?

    P 17   L 21-24

11. What is the great news this book carries to those suffering from alcoholism?

    P 17   L 22-26

WHAT IS THE SOLUTION?

SPIRITUAL EXPERIENCE OR SPIRITUAL AWAKENING CHANGES US

FELLOWSHIP SUPPORTS US

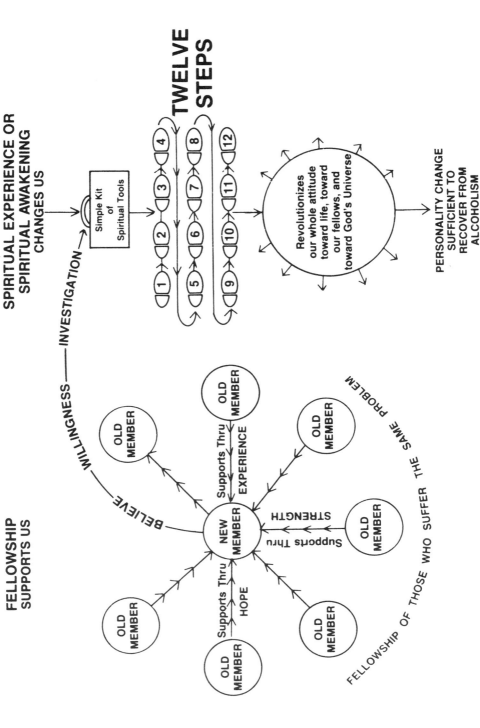

TWELVE STEPS

Simple Kit of Spiritual Tools

WILLINGNESS — INVESTIGATION

Revolutionizes our whole attitude toward life, toward our fellows, and toward God's Universe

PERSONALITY CHANGE SUFFICIENT TO RECOVER FROM ALCOHOLISM

OLD MEMBER

BELIEVE

Supports Thru EXPERIENCE

Supports Thru STRENGTH

Supports Thru HOPE

NEW MEMBER

FELLOWSHIP OF THOSE WHO SUFFER THE SAME PROBLEM

THERE IS A SOLUTION

1. What is alcoholism?
   P 18   L 1-3

2. How are alcoholics treated compared to cancer patients?
   P 18   L 3-11

3. Can this book help the alcoholic family?
   P 18   L 12-13

4. Can the alcoholic talk to medical people?
   P 18   L 14-16

5. Can the alcoholic talk to his family?
   P 18   L 17-19

6. Who can win the confidence of the alcoholic?
   P 18   L 20-24

7. What kind of facts does the recovering alcoholic have?
   P 18   L 21

8. What do these two men have in common?
   P 18   L 26-27

9. What do we have for the new man who has the problem?
   P 18   L 28

10. What is the most effective condition under which we can help the alcoholic?
    P 18   L 29-30

11. How much does our program cost?
    P 18   L 30-31

32 lines on this page

THERE IS A SOLUTION

1. What is the elimination of drinking?
   P 19 L 5-6

2. Where must we practice the AA program?
   P 19 L 6-8

3. Did the early members work with others?
   P 19 L 8-11

4. Is alcoholism a fatal illness?
   P 19 L 14-17

5. Do all alcoholics find help?
   P 19 L 17-18

6. Why did the first 100 give this book to us?
   P 19 L 18-19

7. For whom was this book written?
   P 19 L 20-24

8. Which parts of human life are covered in the book and why?
   P 19 L 25-26

9. Are these subjects controversial?
   P 19 L 26-30

10. How will the AA book handle these subjects?
    P 19 L 30 P 20 L 1

THERE IS A SOLUTION

1. What do the lives of the ex-problem drinkers depend on?
   P 20   L 1-3

2. What question is the reader asking?
   P 20   L 4-10

3. What is the purpose of this book?
   P 20   L 11-13

4. What kind of answers is given for alcoholism in this book?
   P 20   L 11-12

5. How do some nonalcoholic people compare their drinking to ours?
   P 20   L 15-23

6. Does the nonalcoholic understand the alcoholic?
   P 20   L 25-26

7. Does the nonalcoholic react to alcohol like the alcoholic?
   P 20   L 26-28

8. What is the first type of drinker?
   P 20   L 29-31

9. What is the second type of drinker?
   P 20   L 32   P 21   L 7

THERE IS A SOLUTION

1. Does alcohol kill the hard drinker?

   P 21   L 1-2

2. Can the hard drinker quit drinking?

   P 21   L 5

3. What is the third type of drinker?

   P 21   L 8

4. Can he at some point be like the other two types?

   P 21   L 8-12

5. Once a moderate or heavy drinker becomes a real alcoholic, what begins to happen to him?

   P 21   L 11-12

6. What are the two sides of Dr. Jekyll and Mr. Hyde?

   P 21   L 15-end

THERE IS A SOLUTION

1. What does the alcoholic do with his money?
   P 22 L 2-5

2. How do alcoholics get started on other drugs?
   P 22 L 5-7

3. How do alcoholics obtain their drugs?
   P 22 L 9-12

4. What four questions are asked on this page?
   P 22 L 16-22

5. Do we have the answers to those questions?
   P 22 L 23-25

6. What happens when the alcoholic keeps away from a drink?
   P 22 L 28-30

7. What happens when he drinks?
   P 22 L 30 P 23 L 2

THERE IS A SOLUTION

1. Why are observations about the alcoholic academic?

   P 23   L 3-5

2. What is the main problem of the alcoholic?

   P 23   L 5-7

3. If you ask an alcoholic why he started to drink, what answer do you get?

   P 23   L 7-12

4. When you ask an alcoholic about his reason for drinking, what happens?

   P 23   L 15-20

5. Do they know why they took the first drink?

   P 23   L 18-23

6. What is the great obsession of every alcoholic?

   P 23   L 24-26

7. What do families and friends sense?

   P 23   L 27-29

8. What are families and friends waiting for?

   P 23   L 29-31

9. What is the tragic truth?

   P 23   L 32-end

THERE IS A SOLUTION

1. What happens at a certain point?

   P 24   L 1-3

2. Does the drinker know what is happening to him?

   P 24   L 4-5

3. What is the fact about most drinkers who have reached this point?

   P 24   L 6-12

4. Does the alcoholic have a mental defense against the first drink?

   P 24   L 12

5. Does there seem to be a failure of the mental defense?

   P 24   L 18-19

6. What happens when we think about drinking?

   P 24   L 20-22

7. What is the alcoholic beyond?

   P 24   L 29-31

8. What is the alcoholic's future?

   P 24   L 31-32

THERE IS A SOLUTION

1. Did the first 100 like the solution?
   P 25   L 4-7

2. What made these people accept this solution?
   P 25   L 7-13

3. What did the first 100 receive by using the spiritual tools?
   P 25   L 13-15

4. What is the one great fact this book gives?
   P 25   L 16-17

5. What appears at the end of line 17? Follow to bottom of page.
   P 25   L 17

6. What did the spiritual experience do for these people?
   P 25   L 18-19

7. What did the spiritual experience give to the lives of these people?
   P 25   L 20-24

8. Is there a middle-of-the-road solution?
   P 25   L 25-26

9. Where are the first two steps described?
   P 25   L 29-end

SPIRITUAL EXPERIENCE
APPENDIX II

1. What two terms are used in this book?

   P 569   L 1-2

2. What do spiritual experience and spiritual awakening bring about?

   P 569   L 3-4

3. What impression did the reader get from the first Big Book that did not have this?

   P 569   L 6-10

4. What is described in the first few chapters?

   P 569   L 11-12

5. What did the reader of the first book conclude?

   P 569   L 12-17

6. Do some AA members still have this sudden change?

   P 569   L 18-20

7. What kind of changes occur in most AA members?

   P 569   L 20-22

8. How much time is involved in the educational variety experience?

   P 569   L 22-24

9. What does a person realize after having a spiritual experience of the educational variety?

   P 569   L 24-27

10. How long does it take to complete the process?

    P 569   L 27-29

11. After a few months, what do these people find they have accomplished?

    P 569   L 30   P 570   L 2

30 lines on this page

SPIRITUAL EXPERIENCE
APPENDIX II

1. At this time what do they become conscious of?

   P 570   L 3-5

2. What is the only way an alcoholic can fail?

   P 570   L 6-9

3. What is the only thing that can defeat the alcoholic?

   P 570   L 9-10

4. Is there any need for any difficulty with this spiritual program?

   P 570   L 11-12

5. What are the tools needed for recovery?

   P 570   L 12-14

6. What principle can keep us in the darkness of alcoholism?

   P 570   L 15-18

THERE IS A SOLUTION

1. In the story of the man who first received the solution to alcoholism, had he been treated before?

   P 26   L 3-5

2. Had he sought help in this country?

   P 26   L 5-6

3. Where did he then go?

   P 26   L 6-8

4. Whom did he see?

   P 26   L 8

5. Did he finish his treatment?

   P 26   L 10

6. How did he feel after leaving treatment?

   P 26   L 11-12

7. What did he believe?

   P 26   L 12-14

8. What happened?

   P 26   L 15

9. Did he know what made him get drunk?

   P 26   L 15-17

10. Did he go back to treatment?

    P 26   L 18

11. What did he ask the doctor?

    P 26   L 19-25

12. What was the truth the doctor told him?

    P 26   L 25-29

13. Did this man recover?

    P 26   L 30   P 27   L 2

32 lines on this page

THERE IS A SOLUTION

1. Do some alcoholics think they can stay sober without spiritual help?

   P 27   L 3-5

2. What was the doctor's outlook for this man?

   P 27   L 6-9

3. What did the man ask Doctor Jung?

   P 27   L 11

4. Although most alcoholics died or were insane at this time, what was the exception?

   P 27   L 12-16

5. Did this exception occur very often?

   P 27   L 14-15

6. Did Doctor Jung understand this occurrence?

   P 27   L 16

7. What did the exception cause to happen in the alcoholic?

   P 27   L 18-22

8. In this story, where is the psychic change described?

   P 27   L 18-22

9. Had Doctor Jung tried to produce this change?

   P 27   L 22-24

10. Was he successful in producing this change?

    P 27   L 24-25

11. Had he ever been successful in producing one in an alcoholic?

    P 27   L 25-26

12. Can an alcoholic recover from alcoholism on a religious conviction?

    P 27   L 27-end

THERE IS A SOLUTION

1. Did this man have a spiritual experience?
   P 28   L 1-3

2. What did the spiritual experience do for this man?
   P 28   L 3-4

3. Are alcoholics like drowning men?
   P 28   L 5-6

4. When we first get the spiritual experience, what is it like?
   P 28   L 6-7

5. What does this flimsy reed grow into?
   P 28   L 7-8

6. Is there just a single way to approach God?
   P 28   L 10-13

7. Who can find God?
   P 28   L 15-20

8. Is God exclusive?
   P 28   L 15-20

9. Will this spiritual approach interfere with any religious affiliation?
   P 28   L 20-23

10. Does AA care which religious affiliation its members belong to?
    P 28   L 24-28

11. Do all AA members belong to a church?
    P 28   L 28-29

12. What is in chapter 3?
    P 28   L 30-31

13. What is chapter 4 about?
    P 28   L 31-32

14. In what class were many of the first 100?
    P 28   L 32-end

THERE IS A SOLUTION

1. Does being an agnostic block us from a spiritual experience?

   P 29   L 1-2

2. Where is the plan of recovery in the Big Book?

   P 29   L 3-4

3. What else follows the recovery section of the Big Book?

   P 29   L 4-5

4. What will we find in these stories?

   P 29   L 6-8

5. What do we hope these stories will help us do?

   P 29   L 12-17

6. If we identify with these stories, what can be said?

   P 29   L 16-17

WORD DEFINITION
THERE IS A SOLUTION

PAGE 17

CAMARADERIE: good feeling existing between comrades

CAPTAIN'S TABLE: head table

COMMON SOLUTION: the same or shared answer to a problem

PAGE 18

AXES TO GRIND: selfish purposes

ANNIHILATION: destruction

ILLNESS: an unhealthy condition of body or mind

HOLIER THAN THOU: an attitude of feeling superior; spiritually pure

PAGE 19

OBLIVION: being forgotten

PAGE 20

COMMONPLACE: having to do with, belonging to, or used by everybody

PAGE 21

ANTI-SOCIAL: contrary or hostile to the well-being of society

DECISION; a choice

DR. JEKYLL & MR. HYDE: become two different people

GETTING TIGHT: drinking too much

PAGE 22

DEBACLE: complete failure; disaster

MORPHINE: a bitter, white, crystalline, habit-forming drug made from opium

SEDATIVE: a drug that calms or relieves tension

ABNORMAL: not natural

ACADEMIC: not practical; abstract

BENDER: a drinking spree

BAFFLED: confused, bewildered

DOWN FOR THE COUNT: defeated (boxing term)

FALLACIOUS: misleading, delusive (cherish a fallacious hope)

MALADY: disease or disorder of the body or mind; ailment

LETHARGY: abnormal drowsiness; laziness; indifference

PHILOSOPHY: belief, attitude

PLAUSIBILITY: worthiness, reasonableness

ROUSE HIMSELF: to awaken or get active

OBSESSION: a compulsive, often unreasonable idea or feeling

CONSCIOUSNESS: awareness of something

LEGIONS OF ALCOHOLICS: a lot of alcoholics

NONCHALANT: unconcerned, easy

NO AVAIL: no use or advantage

THREAD BARE: shabby

ALTERNATIVES: choices

COUSUMMATION: completion

EXPERIENCE: knowledge or skill gained by actually doing or feeling something

FOURTH DIMENSION: something outside ordinary experience

MIRACULOUS: supernatural; of divine origin

MIDDLE OF THE ROAD: between two extremes

SPIRITUAL: divine

PAGE **26**

A CERTAIN BUSINESS MAN: Roland H.

DR. JUNG: celebrated psychiatrist

POINT-BLANK: clearly, directly

RELAPSE: a return to a former condition after a change for the better

PAGE 27

CONCEPTION: a general idea or understanding

DISPLACEMENT: removal from the usual or proper place

EMOTIONAL: related to feelings

PHENOMENA: things known through the senses but not understood by the mind

REARRANGE: change into a new and proper order

PAGE 28

DESIGN FOR LIVING: way of life

DESPERATION: giving up hope

EXTRAORDINARY: beyond or out of the usual order or method

RELIGIOUS AFFILIATION: one of the systems of faith and worship one is connected or associated with

PAGE 29

OBSTACLE: something that stands in the way of progress toward a goal

CHAPTER 3
MORE ABOUT ALCOHOLISM

1. What is it that most alcoholics are not willing to admit?

   P 30   L 1-2

2. Why is this?

   P 30   L 2-3

3. What one thing does the alcoholic try to prove?

   P 30   L 4-6

4. What is the great obsession of every abnormal drinker?

   P 30   L 6-9

5. Where does this illusion carry the alcoholic?

   P 30   L 9-10

6. To what does the alcoholic have to fully concede?

   P 30   L 11-12

7. What step has the alcoholic taken when he concedes to his innermost self that he is an alcoholic?

   P 30   L 12-13

8. What must we do to this delusion?

   P 30   L 13-14

9. Does the alcoholic ever regain control of this?

   P 30   L 15-21

10. Of what are we convinced?

    P 30   L 21-24

11. What is the alcoholic like?

    P 30   L 25   P 31   L 1

MORE ABOUT ALCOHOLISM

1. Can alcoholics be made into normal drinkers?
   P 31   L 4-7

2. What deception grips the alcoholic?
   P 31   L 8-12

3. What methods have we tried to escape the truth?
   P 31   L 17-29

4. What is the first test we can use to diagnose ourselves?
   P 31   L 30   P 32   L 4

5. How far do we have to travel to take this test?
   P 31   L 31-33

6. Should we try this just once?
   P 31   L 33   P 32   L 1

MORE ABOUT ALCOHOLISM

1. How long will it take to get results from your test?
   P 32   L 1-2

2. Will this test help the alcoholic?
   P 32   L 2-4

3. When can the alcoholic stop drinking?
   P 32   L 5-7

4. Why don't alcoholics quit when they can?
   P 32   L 7-9

5. Where is the point of insanity in this story?
   P 32   L 23-26

32 lines on this page

MORE ABOUT ALCOHOLISM

1. What was the result, insanity or death?
   P 33   L 2-3

2. What insane idea have we believed?
   P 33   L 4-6

3. What is the real truth?
   P 33   L 8-10

4. What reservation must go if we are to stop drinking?
   P 33   L 12-14

5. How can young people be misled?
   P 33   L 15-23

6. Do you have to drink a long time to become an alcoholic?
   P 33   L 24-26

7. Can women become alcoholics sooner than men?
   P 33   L 26-28

8. How can you insult an alcoholic?
   P 33   L 29-31

32 lines on this page

MORE ABOUT ALCOHOLISM

1. What do we alcoholics see when we are looking back?

   P 34   L 2-4

2. What is the second test given for alcoholism?

   P 34   L 4-6

3. What are his chances of passing this test?

   P 34   L 6-7

4. Can the alcoholic stop for a year?

   P 34   L 7-13

5. Can those who stop still be alcoholics?

   P 34   L 10-11

6. Can those who come to the point where they read the Big Book stop for a year?

   P 34   L 12-13

7. What is baffling about alcoholism?

   P 34   L 24-26

31 lines on this page

MORE ABOUT ALCOHOLISM

1. What is the crux of the problem?
   P 35   L 1-3

2. What two questions do the friends of the alcoholic ask?
   P 35   L 4-10

3. How old was Jim when he took his first drink?
   P 35   L 16-17

4. How did he begin to act when drinking?
   P 35   L 17-19

5. Where did he sober up?
   P 35   L 19

6. Which two steps did the first 100 tell him about?
   P 35   L 21-22

7. Step 3 is a beginning. Did he take step 3?
   P 35   L 22

8. He went to work and did well, but did he build on the first three steps?
   P 35   L 25-26

9. Did the sober members of AA give up on this man?
   P 35   L 27-29

10. Did he agree to stop?
    P 35   L 29-30

11. Did he know what drinking would cause?
    P 35   L 30-31

MORE ABOUT ALCOHOLISM

1. Why was Jim irritated?

   P 36   L 3-6

2. What were his intentions?

   P 36   L 6-7

3. Did he go to the bar to drink?

   P 36   L 7-11

4. What was his first order?

   P 36   L 14-15

5. What was his second order?

   P 36   L 16-17

6. What happened before his third order?

   P 36   L 18-20

7. What was his third order?

   P 36   L 20-21

8. Did he sense he was doing something wrong?

   P 36   L 21-22

9. What was his fourth order?

   P 36   L 23-24

10. Was there a fifth order?

    P 36   L 25-26

11. Did he end up in the same place?

    P 36   L 27-28

12. Did he know he was an alcoholic?

    P 36   L 31-32

13. What foolish idea pushed aside the fact that he was an alcoholic?

    P 36   L 32   P 37   L 1

32 lines on this page

MORE ABOUT ALCOHOLISM

1. What do we call this kind of thinking?

   P 37   L 3-4

2. What is insanity?

   P 37   L 4-6

3. Have we all thought like this?

   P 37   L 7-9

4. What overrode our sound reasoning?

   P 37   L 11-14

5. The next day what would we ask ourselves?

   P 37   L 15-17

6. When we did deliberately drink, did we stop to think before we drank?

   P 37   L 18-24

7. In the second story, what is the obsession for drinking compared to?

   P 37   L 28-30

8. Does he enjoy his jay-walking life the way we did our early years of drinking?

   P 37   L 31-end

MORE ABOUT ALCOHOLISM

1. Does this problem start small?
   P 38   L 1-3

2. Is this man normal?
   P 38   L 3

3. Does his problem get worse?
   P 38   L 4-6

4. Did he decide to quit on his own?
   P 38   L 6-7

5. Did he stay quit?
   P 38   L 8

6. Did he quit again?
   P 38   L 9-11

7. Did he lose that ability to earn a living like some alcoholics?
   P 38   L 11-12

8. Did his wife react like the wife of an alcoholic?
   P 38   L 12

9. Is the main problem of this man in his body or his head?
   P 38   L 13-14

10. Does he quit the third time?
    P 38   L 14-15

11. Does it work? What happens?
    P 38   L 15-17

12. What conclusion can be made of this man?
    P 38   L 17-18

13. Is this a little like the alcoholic? Is he exactly like the alcoholic?
    P 38   L 19-22

MORE ABOUT ALCOHOLISM

14. Is the alcoholic an intelligent person in other matters?

    P 38   L 22-25

15. Where is he insane?

    P 38   L 23-25

16. What excuse do people make who think they are a little bit of an alcoholic?

    P 38   L 27   P 39   L 1-2

32 lines on this page

MORE ABOUT ALCOHOLISM

1. Can the alcoholic stay sober on self-knowledge?

   P 39   L 7-9

2. Is this point important to the life of the alcoholic?

   P 39   L 9-13

3. Our next story explains again the state of mind that precedes the first drink. Where did Fred sober up?

   P 39   L 21-23

4. Would Fred take the first step like Jim?

   P 39   L 23-33

5. Did he quit drinking like the jay-walker quit jay-walking?

   P 39   L 28-29

6. Would he take step 1 or did he want to stop drinking on his own?

   P 39   L 31   P 40   L 7

7. Did they talk to Fred about the first step?

   P 39   L 33   P 40   L 1

MORE ABOUT ALCOHOLISM

1. Did Fred think he was a little alcoholic?

   P 40   L 1-4

2. When Fred got drunk and went back to the hospital, was he ready to listen?

   P 40   L 8-11

3. What made him reject the first step?

   P 40   L 16-28

4. Did he think quitting was a simple matter?

   P 40   L 29-32

MORE ABOUT ALCOHOLISM

1. How was Fred's life going when his insantiy started? Was he irritated and down in the dumps like Jim in the first story?

   P 41   L 1-7

2. With everything going good, what insane idea came to his head?

   P 41   L 8-11

3. What did the physical craving cause him to do after the first drink?

   P 41   L 12-24

4. How well did his will power do in combatting the power of obsession?

   P 41   L 26-29

MORE ABOUT ALCOHOLISM

1. What did they tell him about will power?

   P 42   L 1-3

2. What did Jim realize was wrong with his mind?

   P 42   L 5-8

3. When is it that will power will not work?

   P 42   L 6-8

4. Could Fred then identify with other recovered alcoholics on the first step?

   P 42   L 8-10

5. Did other things help him take the first step 100%?

   P 42   L 11-20

6. Did they give him step 2 and the 10 steps of action?

   P 421   L 21-23

7. Was the program of recovery easy for Fred?

   P 42   L 23-31

8. What solved all of Fred's problems?

   P 42   L 32-end

MORE ABOUT ALCOHOLISM

1. What did Fred find in the program?

   P 43   L 1-6

2. Was Fred a chronic alcoholic?

   P 43   L 7-11

3. Do doctors and psychiatrists agree that alcoholism is a hopeless condition?

   P 43   L 12-17

4. Is the alcoholic hopeless without divine help?

   P 43   L 17-19

5. Is there any solution for alcoholics other than a spiritual experience?

   P 43   L 18-25

6. The story of Fred and Jim and this complete chapter make one main point to the reader. What is that point?

   P 43   L 26-end

WORD DEFINITION
MORE ABOUT ALCOHOLISM

PAGE 30
OBSESSION: a compulsive, often unreasonable idea or feeling

ABNORMAL: not natural

ILLUSION: something that misleads or deceives

CONCEDE: acknowledge as true; admit

DELUSION: a false belief held as a result of self-deception

INSANITY: not whole of mind

INCOMPREHENSIBLE: incapable of being understood

DEMORALIZATION: discouragement

PAGE 31
REMEDY: a cure

DECEPTION: a state of being misled

INABILITY: lack of means or ability

SOLEMN OATH: serious promise to fulfill a pledge

SANITARIUM: a place for the care of the chronically ill

ASYLUM: an institution for the care of the mentally ill

ABRUPTLY: suddenly

PAGE 32
HUMILIATED: lowered in pride, dignity or status; disgraced

PAGE 33
LURKING: lying in ambush; hidden

PAGE 34
SCANT: meager or inadequate

POTENTIAL: capable of being but not yet in existence

ASSUMING: taking to be true
BAFFLING: bewildering, confusing

PAGE 35

PRECEDE: go in advance of; go before

RELAPSE: a return to a former condition after a change for the better

CRUX: basic or essential thing

REASONED: thought logically

SPREE: drinking bout
CONSTERNATION: sudden confusion, amazement or frustration

PAGE 36
VAGUELY: not clearly

COMMITMENT: forced confinement

PAGE 37
PREMEDITATION: plotting in advance

ABSURD: ridiculous, unreasonable

PAGE 38
CHAP: man, fellow

RIDICULE: make fun of

CRAZY: insane

PAGE 39
INTIMATED: hinted

DEPRESSED: in low spirits; dejected

PAGE 41
LANDING FIELD: where planes land

PROPHESIED: predicted

PAGE 42
NOMINAL: not in practice but in name only

CHAPTER 4
WE AGNOSTICS

1. What are the two questions one must ask himself to determine if he is an alcoholic?

   P 44   L 4-7

2. What is the only solution to alcoholism?

   P 44   L 7-9

3. Does this seem impossible for the atheist or agnostic?

   P 44   L 10-15

4. How many of the original fellowship thought a spiritual experience impossible?

   P 44   L 16-17

5. What fact did we have to face?

   P 22   L 19-21

6. How many of us thought we were atheists or agnostics?

   P 44   L 22-23

7. Will a code of morals or a better philosophy of life over-come alcoholism?

   P 44   L 25   P 45   L 3

WE AGNOSTICS

1. How had our power and our will worked?
   P 45   L 3-8

2. What was our dilemma?
   P 45   L 9

3. What did we have to find?
   P 45 L 9-11

4. What is the main object of this book?
   P 45   L 13-15

5. What kind of book is this?
   P 45   L 15-17

6. What is this book going to talk about?
   P 45   L 17-18

7. What happens to the new man when we talk about God?
   P 45   L 18-25

8. What did we think about the idea of God dependence?
   P 45   L 33   P 46   L 3

WE AGNOSTICS

1. What turned us off from God?

   P 46   L 3-9

2. Where could we see God at work?

   P 46   L 9-11

3. What happened when we laid aside prejudice and expressed a willingness to believe?

   P 46   L 15-20

4. What did we discover about other people's conception of God?

   P 46   L 21-24

5 What did we have to do to have this power?

   P 46   L 25-28

6. Does God drive a hard bargain?

   P 46   L 29-30

7. Is God exclusive?

   P 46   L 30-32

8. Who is open to God?

   P 46   L 33

WE AGNOSTICS

1. When we speak to you of God, what do we mean?

   P 47   L 1-2

2. What must we ask ourselves about spiritual terms in order to commence growth?

   P 47   L 4-9

3. Where did we begin?

   P 47   L 11-13

4. What question did we need to ask ourselves?

   P 47   L 14-16

5. As soon as we believe, what happens?

   P 47   L 16-19

6. What are we building in order to stay sober?

   P 47   L 19-21

7. What did the first 100 think was needed to start?

   P 47   L 22-25

8. Did they want the faith of others?

   P 47   L 25-27

9. What did they learn that was comforting?

   P 47   L 30-31

WE AGNOSTICS

1. Besides a lack of faith, what other handicaps did we have in this area?

   P 48   L 1-4

2. What had to be done with this sort of thinking?

   P 48   L 4-5

3. How did we become open-minded on spiritual matters?

   P 48   L 7-11

4. What does the practical individual of today demand?

   P 48   L 17-18

5. On what condition do we accept theories?

   P 48   L 18-20

6. Why does everyone accept, for example, the theories about electricity?

   P 48   L 20-25

7. Upon what does everybody base their assumptions nowadays?

   P 48   L 26-28

8. What does science demonstrate?

   P 48   L 28-29

9. As mankind studies the material world, what is being revealed?

   P 48   L 29-32

10. How does science describe the "prosaic steel gird⌐

    P 48   L 33   P 49   L 1

WE AGNOSTICS

1. Do we doubt it?

   P 49   L 4

2. When the idea of God is suggested, how do we react?

   P 49   L 4-12

3. What if there were no God?

   P 49   L 12-14

4. What did we agnostics and atheists believe?

   P 49   L 15-20

5. What do we beg of you?

   P 49   L 21-22

6. What have we learned about people of faith?

   P 49   L 23-26

7. What was our conception of life?

   P 49   L 26-27

8. How did we amuse ourselves, and what didn't we observe?

   P 49   L 27-end

WE AGNOSTICS

1. On what basis did we condemn and justify our intolerance of these people of faith?

   P 50   L 1-4

2. What did we miss as the result of being unfair about spiritual matters?

   P 50   L 4-7

3. What will you find in our personal stories?

   P 50   L 8-10

4. Must we all agree with a particular approach or conception?

   P 50   L 10-15

5. What is the one proposition upon which we all agree?

   P 50   L 16-22

6. What do thousands of worldly men and women declare as the reason for the revolutionary change in their way of living and thinking?

   P 50   L 23-28

7. Under what circumstances did they find their new power?

   P 50   L 28-32

8. When did this happen?

   P 50   L 32-33

9. What do their stories show us?

   P 50   L 33   P 51   L 5

WE AGNOSTICS

1. What is the powerful reason presented why one should have faith?

   P 51   L 5-9

2. Have we made more material progress in our lifetime than the men who lived before us?

   P 51   L 10-12

3. Are we more intelligent?

   P 51   L 13-14

4. Why was material progress slow in ancient times?

   P 51   L 15-19

5. How were the ideas of Columbus and Galileo received?

   P 51   L 19-22

6. How do some of us compare to the ancients?

   P 51   L 23-25

7. Why were American newspapers afraid to print the account of the Wright brothers' Kittyhawk flight?

   P 51   L 28   P 52   L 1

WE AGNOSTICS

1. What was commonplace 30 years later?

   P 52   L 1-3

2. What has our generation witnessed in most fields?

   P 52   L 4-5

3. Group Question: Where are we now in space travel in the present year?

   P 52   L 5-8

4. What is characteristic of our age?

   P 52   L 8-12

5. What did we ask ourselves about our human problems?

   P 52   L 13-15

6. What were some of these problems?

   P 52   L 15-23

7. When did we stop doubting the power of God?

   P 52   L 24-27

8. What was the mainspring of the Wright brothers' accomplishment?

   P 52   L 28-31

9. When did we agnostics and atheists change our ideas about self-sufficiency solving our problems?

   P 52   L 31   P 53   L 2

WE AGNOSTICS

1. Is our logic good?
   P 53   L 3-6

2. Is it by accident that man has logic?
   P 53   L 3-4

3. What is the correct use of our logic?
   P 53   L 5-7

4. If it is beyond our logic, will we accept it?
   P 53   L 7-9

5. Is it more logical to believe than not to believe?
   P 53   L 9-14

6. What proposition did we alcoholics have to face?
   P 53   L 15-19

7. Do we have a decision?
   P 53   L 19

8. What confronts us at the turning point?
   P 53   L 20-21

9. Where does reason carry us?
   P 53   L 22-23

10. What do we find in the new land of recovery?
    P 53   L 23-26

11. Why can't we get the shores of faith on firm reasoning?
    P 53   L 26-30

12. What kind of faith had brought us to where we stood?
    P 53   L 31   P 54   L 3

WE AGNOSTICS

1. What had we been faithful to?
   P 54   L 3-6

2. Have we been worshipers?
   P 54   L 7

3. What have we worshiped?
   P 54   L 9-12

4. Have we had love?
   P 54   L 12-13

5. How much pure reason had been involved?
   P 54   L 13-15

6. How important had these feelings been?
   P 54   L 15-18

7. What was impossible to say?
   P 54   L 18-19

8. What had we been living by?
   P 54   L 20-21

9. What would life be based on pure reason?
   P 54   L 22-23

10. Can we prove life by reason?
    P 54   L 24-26

11. Could we say the universe just happened by accident?
    P 54   L 26-31

WE AGNOSTICS

1. Is reason entirely dependable?

   P 54   L 32   P 55   L 2

2. Can reason prove a lie?

   P 55   L 1-2

3. What had we thought about spiritual liberation in others?

   P 55   L 3-8

4. Why were we fooling ourselves?

   P 55   L 9-11

5. Where is God?

   P 55   L 9-11

6. What can cover up this idea?

   P 55   L 11-13

7. How long has he been there?

   P 55   L 13-15

8. What is God?

   P 55   L 16-18

9. How did we find Him?

   P 55   L 18-19

10. Where did we find Him?

    P 55   L 20-22

11. What three things do we hope our testimony has helped you do?

    P 55   L 23-26

12. What can you do then?

    P 55   L 26-27

13. What can you expect with this attitude?

    P 55   L 27-29

14. What story is used to illustrate what we have been describing?

    P 55   L 30-end

WE AGNOSTICS

1. What was his spiritual background?

   P 56   L 1

2. Where did he rebel at religion?

   P 56   L 1-3

3. What sort of troubles did he have?

   P 56   L 3-10

4. Who brought him the message that enabled him to believe?

   P 56   L 11-13

5. What was his reaction to this message?

   P 56   L 13-15

6. Where did he use his logic correctly?

   P 56   L 15-17

7. To what depth did his logic carry him?

   P 56   L 17-19

8. Where did he use his reasoning correctly?

   P 56   L 19-21

9. To what conviction did this decision carry him?

   P 56   L 22-24

10. What was the result of stepping from the bridge of reason to the shores of faith?

    P 56   L 28-30

11. Did this man recover?

    P 56   L 31   P 57   L 5

WE AGNOSTICS

1. What is this?

   P 57   L 6

2. Is the recovery program complicated?

   P 57   L 6-7

3. Did circumstances enable him to take step 2?

   P 57   L 7-8

4. Did step 2 enable him to take step 3?

   P 57   L 8-9

5. Did this man have a spiritual experience or a spiritual awakening?

   P 57   L 10-11

6. Do we all have a sudden spiritual experience?

   P 57   L 11-13

7. Can anyone who honestly seeks God fail to find Him?

   P 57   L 12-13

8. What do we have to do for God to disclose Himself to us?

   P 57   L 14-15

WORD DEFINITION
WE AGNOSTICS

PAGE 44

PRECEDING: going before; going in advance of

CONQUER: to overcome or be victorious

ATHEIST: one who denies the existence of God

AGNOSTIC: one who believes that God is unknown and probably unknowable

DOOMED: condemned to an unhappy destiny

BASIS: basic principle

ALTERNATIVES: choices

DISCONCERTED: thrown into confusion

MORALS: teachings governing right thought and behavior

PHILOSOPHY: overall vision or attitude

PAGE 45

MARSHALLED: brought together

WILL: strong desire

SUFFICIENT: enough to meet the needs of a situation

UTTERLY: complete, total, absolute

DILEMMA: unsatisfactory alternative

OBVIOUSLY: easily seen

EVADED: avoided facing up to

ANTI-RELIGIOUS: opposed to religion

PAGE 46

COWARDLY: lacking courage

THEOLOGICAL: the study of God and of religious beliefs

INEXPLICABLE: incapable of being explained

CALAMITY: a major misfortune or loss; disaster

PAGE 48

ELECTRICITY: power of an undetermined origin consisting of negative and positive composed respectively of electrons and protons

MURMUR: soft or low sound

DOUBT: distrust

ASSUMPTION: taken for granted

STARTING POINT: where work or activity begins

BELIEVES: accepts as true or real

VISUAL PROOF: evidence that can be seen

PROSAIC: dull, unimaginative

STEEL GIRDER: a horizontal part of a structure that supports a vertical load

PAGE 49

LABORIOUSLY: with great effort

INDULGE: take pleasure in

WINDY: lacking substance

INTELLIGENCE: knowledge

ALPHA: beginning; first letter in Greek alphabet

OMEGA: end; last letter in Greek alphabet

DUBIOUS: questionable, doubtful

ORGANIZED RELIGION: coordinated worship

FRAILTIES: weaknesses

LOGICAL: reasonable, valid

CYNICALLY: distrustfully

DISSECTING: separating into pieces; cutting apart

STABILITY: not changing; steadiness

SHORTCOMINGS: deficiencies, flaws, faults

CONDEMNATION: blame

INTOLERANCE: unwillingness to allow or respect the beliefs or behavior of others

DIVERTED: turned aside

MIRACULOUS: supernatural; of divine origin

BAFFLED: confused, bewildered

MILLENNIUMS: periods of 1,000 years

INTELLECT: capacity for knowledge

REALM: possibility of

FETTERED: hampered

SUPERSTITION: a belief or practice resulting from ignorance

TRADITION: information, beliefs and customs handed down by each generation to the next

CONTEMPORARIES: people the same or nearly the same age

COLUMBUS: Christopher Columbus (1451-1506). Italian navigator who discovered America

PREPOSTEROUS: absurd

GALILEO: Galileo Galilei, founder of astronomy

ASTRONOMICAL: relating to the stars, planets and other bodies in the sky

HERESIES: opinions contrary to accepted beliefs

BIASED: prejudiced

WRIGHT BROTHERS: Orville (1871-1948) and Wilbur (1867-1912). American pioneers in aviation

PAGE 53
DUCK: avoid, evade

LUSTRE: shine, glow

FLAGGING: weak, dwindling

PAGE 54
BELIEVE: accept as true or real

REASONING: ability to think

WORSHIPERS: people showing extravagant respect

MENTAL GOOSE-FLESH: state of fear

MOTIVE: need or desire that causes one to act

FAITH: trust

MASS OF ELECTRONS: a group of particles charged with negative electricity

PAGE 55
EMANATE: come out of a source

LIBERATION: release

FUNDAMENTAL: basic or primary

MAKE-UP: the way something is put together

ANALYSIS: a critical examination

TESTIMONY: open acknowledgement

PREJUDICE: resentments handed down

DILIGENTLY: using steady effort

BROAD HIGHWAY: a wide, open, all-inclusive course or way

ATTITUDE: mental position or state of mind

CONSCIOUSNESS: awareness

REBELLIOUS: defiant, opposing

OVERDOSE OF RELIGION: excessive or forced religious training

DOGGED: faltering

CALAMITIES: major misfortunes or losses; disasters

EMBITTERED: made bitterly resentful

DISILLUSIONMENT: disenchantment; disappointment

CONVICTION: strong belief

MAJESTY: authority

BARRIERS: things that impede or separate

COMPANIONSHIP: fellowship

CORNERSTONE: foundation

VICISSITUDE: any of one's ups and downs

TEMPTATION: being lured to do wrong

REVULSION: strong distaste

MIRACLE: divine intervention in human affairs

REVELATION: communicating divine truth; something revealed by God to man

CHAPTER FIVE
HOW IT WORKS

Rarely have we seen a person fail who has thoroughly followed our directions. Those who do not recover are people who cannot or will not completely give themselves to this simple program, usually men and women who are constitutionally incapable of being honest with themselves. There are such unfortunates. They are not at fault; they seem to have been born that way. They are naturally incapable of grasping and developing a way of life which demands rigorous honesty. Their chances are less than average. There are those, too, who suffer from grave emotional and mental disorders, but many of them do recover if they have the capacity to be honest.

Our stories disclose in a general way what we used to be like, what happened, and what we are like now. If you have decided you want what we have and are willing to go to any length to get it—then you are ready to follow directions.

At some of these you may balk. You may think you can find an easier, softer way. We doubt if you can. With all the earnestness at our command, we beg of you to be fearless and thorough from the very start. Some of us have tried to hold on to our old ideas and the result was nil until we let go absolutely.

Remember that you are dealing with alcohol—cunning, baffling, powerful! Without help it is too much for you. But there is One who has all power—that One is God. You must find Him now!

Half measures will avail you nothing. You stand at the turning point. Throw yourself under His protection and care with complete abandon.

Now we think you can take it! Here are the steps we took, which are suggested as your Program of Recovery:

1. Admitted we were powerless over alcohol—that our lives had become unmanageable.

2. Came to believe that a Power greater than ourselves could restore us to sanity.

3. Made a decision to turn our will and our lives over to the care and direction of God as we understood Him.

4. Made a searching and fearless moral inventory of ourselves.

5. Admitted to God, to ourselves, and to another human being the exact nature of our wrongs.

6. Were entirely willing that God remove all these defects of character.

7. Humbly, on our knees, asked Him to remove our shortcomings—holding nothing back.

8. Made a list of all persons we had harmed, and became willing to make complete amends to them all.

9. Made direct amends to such people wherever possible, except when to do so would injure them or others.

10. Continued to take personal inventory and when we were wrong promptly admitted it.

11. Sought through prayer and meditation to improve our contact with God, praying only for knowledge of His will for us and the power to carry that out.

12. Having had a spiritual experience as the result of this course of action, we tried to carry this message to others, especially alcoholics, and to practice these principles in all our affairs.

You may exclaim, "What an order! I can't go through with it." Do not be discouraged. No one among us has been able to maintain anything like perfect adherence to these principles. We are not saints. The point is, that we are willing to grow along spiritual lines. The principles we have set down are guides to progress. We claim spiritual progress rather than spiritual perfection.

Our description of the alcoholic, the chapter to the agnostic, and our personal adventures before and after, have been designed to sell you three pertinent ideas:

(a) That you are alcoholic and cannot manage your own life.

(b) That probably no human power can relieve your alcoholism.

(c) That God can and will.

If you are not convinced on these vital issues, you ought to reread the book to this point or else throw it away!

If you are convinced, you are now at step three, which is that you make a decision to turn your will and your life over to God as you understand Him. Just what do we mean by that, and just what do we do?

*The twelve steps from the Book AA are used with the permission of the General Service Office of Alcoholics Anonymous in New York City.

CHAPTER 5
HOW IT WORKS

1. How often do alcoholics fail to recover using the path of the first 100?

   P 58   L 1-2

2. What two kinds of people do not recover in AA?

   P 58   L 2-6

3. How did they become as they are?

   P 58   L 7-8

4. Do they have a 50-50 chance?

   P 58   L 10

5. Does the recovery program work for people who have mental and emotional disorders?

   P 58   L 11-13

6. What three important ideas will our stories disclose?

   P 58   L 14-15

7. How far must one be willing to go to be ready to take the steps?

   P 58   L 16-17

8. Did the first 100 people look forward to taking the steps?

   P 58   L 19-20

9. Did they hunt for an easy way out?

   P 58   L 19-20

10. What did they try to do?

    P 58   L 22-23

11. What were the results?

    P 58   L 23-24

12. What kind of problem does the alcoholic face?

    P 58   L 25   P 59   L 1

 25 lines on this page.

HOW IT WORKS

1. Where does all power come from?

   P 59   L 2   _GOD_

2. Are there several ways that an alcoholic can recover?

   P 59   L 2-3   _NO –_

3. What do we get from half the program?

   P 59   L 4   _NOTHING_

4. At what critical point has the recovered alcoholic stood?

   P 59   L 4-5   _TURNING POINT_

5. How had they asked for his care?

   P 59   L 5-6   _ASKED WITH COMPLETE ABANDON_

READER READS THE 12 STEPS

32 lines on this page.

HOW IT WORKS

1. What opinion did the first alcoholics have when they approached the steps?

   P 60   L 5-6

2. What message do they give to those who follow?

   P 60   L 6-12

3. Where do they mention the following?
   Doctor's Opinion   P 60   L 13
   Chapter 4   P 60   L 13-14
   Bill's Story   P 60   L 14

4. These early chapters show us step 1 and step 2, which make clear what ideas?

   P 60   L 16-20

5. If we are convinced of the fact that we are powerless over alcohol and that there is a power that could relieve our alcoholism, where are we?

   P 60   L 21

6. What is step 3?

   P 60   L 21-24

7. What is the first requirement?

   P 60   L 25-26

8. What happens to people who try to live on self-will?

   P 60   L 26-28

9. Is the alcoholic the only person who tries to live on self-will?

   P 60   L 29

10. What are people like who live on self-propulsion?

    P 60   L 29   P 61   L 10

32 lines on this page.

HOW IT WORKS

1. Does the actor get along well?

   P 61   L 11-12

2. When this does not work, does he change what does he do?

   P 61   L 12-15

3. Does he like the play?

   P 61   L 15

4. Whom does the actor running the show blame?

   P 61   L 16-17

5. Does he develop a bad attitude?

   P 61   L 17-18

6. What is his basic trouble?

   P 61   L 18-20

7. What is he a victim of?

   P 61   L 20-22   DELUSION

8. What can the other players plainly see?

   P 61   L 22-24

9. What does his action do to the rest of the players?

   P 61   L 24-26

10. At his best, what does the actor produce?

    P 61   L 26-27

HOW IT WORKS

1. What are most people in this state of mind concerned about?

   P 62   L 3-5

2. What is the root problem?

   P 62   L 6-7

3. What does this cause him and others to do?

   P 62   L 7-9

4. What causes others to hurt us?

   P 62   L 9-13

5. Who makes our trouble?

   P 62   L 14-15

6. The alcoholic is an example of what?

   P 62   L 15-17

7. What has he got to get rid of?

   P 62   L 17-18

8. If he keeps it, what will happen?

   P 62   L 18-19

9. How does he get rid of it?

   P 62   L 19

10. Is this the only way?

    P 62   L 19-21

11. Have we used everything else trying to get rid of it?

    P 62   L 21-25

12. What is the only answer?

    P 62   L 25

13. What have we been playing and why should we quit doing this?

    P 62   L 26-27

14. How have we decided to live in the future?

    P 62   L 27-30

HOW IT WORKS

15. What stone is step 3 in the arch to freedom?

    P 62   L 32

HOW IT WORKS

1. What are the results of taking step 3?
   P 63   L 1-12

2. How did many of the first 100 take step 3?
   P 63   L 13-22

3. Did the first 100 take step 3 by themselves?
   P 63   L 23-25

4. Can step 3 be taken alone?
   P 63   L 25-26

5. Do we need certain words in prayer to find God?
   P 63   L 26-28

6. Do we get a lot of results from step 3?
   P 63   L 29-31

7. After we finish step 3, what do we do?
   P 63   L 32-end

HOW IT WORKS

1. What was step 3?

   P 64   L 1-2

2. Do we recover with step 3?

   P 64   L 2-3

3. When should we take step 4?

   P 64   L 3

4. Is there something in ourselves that is blocking us from our decision in step 3?

   P 64   L 4-5

5. Does alcohol help us live with these things?

   P 64   L 5-6

6. Do they have to be dealt with?

   P 64   L 6-7

7. Our personal inventory is compared to what kind of inventory?

   P 64   L 8-10

8. Our searching and fearless inventory is compared to what?

   P 64   L 10-11

9. What is an inventory?

   P 64   L 11-13

10. If our lives are a business, what do we have to do?

    P 64   L 13-16

11. What did we do about our failing business?

    P 64   L 17-22

HOW IT WORKS

12. What are the instructions for filling out the inventory on page 64?

    P 64   L 23-33

13. What is it in the first column we are asked to fill out from top to bottom?

    P 64   L 29-30

14. What do we put in the second column?

    P 64   L 31

15. What do we put in the third column?

    P 64   L 31   P 65   L 2

HOW IT WORKS

1. Where are these instructions for taking the inventory repeated on page 65?

   P 65   L 3-6

2. The reader should read the list of people in the first column (I am resentful at) in the inventory examples.

3. The next reader should read the second column (the cause).

4. The next reader should read the third column (which part of self was affected by the resentment).

Do not work the inventory from left to right. This would require the mind to look at three things at the same time. Fill in each column from top to bottom completely before going on to the next column.

5. Where do we apply this example?

   P 65   L 31

6. What counts?

   P 65   L 31-32

7. When we finish our resentment inventory, what do we do with it?

   P 65   L 32-33

8. What is the first theory we learn when we first see our list of resentments on paper?

   P 65   L 33   P 66   L 2

HOW IT WORKS

1. Have we done this before?

    P 66   L 2-3

2. Did this make us sore?

    P 66   L 3-6

3. When we fought, did things get better?

    P 66   L 6-7

4. Did we ever win?

    P 66   L 7-9

5. What is the second thing we can see in our resentment inventory?

    P 66   L 10-11

6. In the resentment inventory, what do we find we have been wasting?

    P 66   L 11-13

7. All these other things are bad, but what is the worst thing resentment can cause?

    P 66   L 13-16

8. What happens to the alcoholic who harbors resentment?

    P 66   L 16-19

9. If we are to live, who do we have to be free of?

    P 66   L 20-21

10. Can other people have resentment?

    P 66   L 21-22

11. What is resentment for the alcoholic?

    P 66   L 22-23

12. What does our resentment list hold?   *The key to (the) our future.*

    P 66   L 24-25

HOW IT WORKS

13. We learned that while in resentment, what did we allow other people to do?

    P 66   L 27-29

14. After seeing all of this, what must we now do?

    P 66   L 29-31

15. Can we wish resentment away?

    P 66   L 30-31

16. What is the first thing we do?

    P 66   L 32   P 67   L 2

REVIEW OF FEARS

INSTRUCTIONS FOR COMPLETION

Instruction 1 In dealing with fears we put them on paper. We listed people, institutions or principles with whom we were fearful. (Complete Column 1 from top to bottom. Do nothing on Columns 2, 3 or 4 until Column 1 is complete.)

Instruction 2 We asked ourselves why do I have the fear. (Complete Column 2 from top to bottom. Do nothing on Columns 3 or 4 until Column 2 is complete.)

Instruction 3 Which part of self caused the fear. Was it our self esteem, our security, our ambitions, our personal or sex relations which had been interfered with? (Complete each column within Column 3 going from top to bottom. Start-ing with the Self-Esteem Column and finishing with the Sexual Ambitions Column. Do nothing on Column 4 until Column 3 is complete.)

Instruction 4 Referring to our list again. Putting out of our minds the wrongs others had done, we resolutely looked for our own mistakes. Where had we been selfish, dishonest, self-seeking and frightened and inconsiderate? (Asking our-selves the above questions we complete each column within Column 4.)

Instruction 5 Reading from left to right we now see the fear (Column 1), why do I have the fear (Column 2), the part of self that caused the fear (Column 3), and the exact nature of the defect within us that allowed the fear to surface and block us off from God's will (Column 4).

	COLUMN 1 I'm fearful of:	COLUMN 2 Why do I have the fear?	COLUMN 3 "SELF" AFFECTS MY (Which part of self caused the Fear?)										COLUMN 4 What is the exact nature of my wrongs, faults, mistakes, defects, shortcomings:			
			Social Instinct		Security Instinct		Sex Instinct		Ambitions			Selfish	Dishonest	Self-Seeking & Frightened	Inconsiderate	
			Self-Esteem	Personal Relationships	Material	Emotional	Acceptable Sex Relations	Hidden Sex Relations	Social	Security	Sexual					
1																
2																
3																
4																
5																
6																
7																
8																

4-B

HOW IT WORKS

1. Why do they hurt us?
   P 67   L 1-2

2. Where is the fourth step prayer?
   P 67   L 3-8

3. What is the third thing we must learn to do?
   P 67   L 9-13

4. What goes in the fourth column of our inventory?
   P 67   L 14-24

5. After resentment, what do we look at next?
   P 67   L 25-27

6. Do alcoholics have fear?
   P 67   L 27-30

7. What does it do to them?
   P 67   L 30-31

8. Who started the fear?
   P 67   L 31-end

32 lines on this page.

HOW IT WORKS

1. What is fear like and what does it do to us?

   P 68   L 1-2

2. What do we do about our fears?

   P 68   L 3

3. Do we list them as we did our resentments?

   P 68   L 3-5

4. What goes in the second column?

   P 68   L 5-6

5. What caused our fears?

   P 68   L 6

6. What do we do?

   P 68   L 13-14

7. After we see what our fears have been doing to us, what do we do in the future?

   P 68   L 14-15

8. What will come as the result of our new plans?

   P 68   L 15-17

9. Is this the way of weakness?

   P 68   L 19-23

10. What can God do with our lives?

    P 68   L 23-24

11. Where is the prayer that deals with fear?

    P 68   L 24-26

12. What happens at once when we use this prayer?

    P 68   L 26-27

13. What is the last part of self to be mentioned?

    P 68   L 28

HOW IT WORKS

14. What do we need in our sex lives?

    P 68   L 28-29

15. How are we going to approach this subject?

    P 68   L 29-30

16. Do people have different views on this subject?

    P 68   L 30   P 69   L 6

REVIEW OF RESENTMENTS
INSTRUCTIONS FOR COMPLETION

Instruction 1 In dealing with resentments we set them on paper. We listed people, institutions or principles with whom we were angry. (Complete Column 1 from top to bottom. Do nothing on Columns 2, 3 or 4 until Column 1 is complete.)

Instruction 2 We asked ourselves why we were angry. (Complete Column 2 from top to bottom. Do nothing on Columns 3 or 4 until Column 2 is complete.)

Instruction 3 On our grudge list we set opposite each name our injuries. Was it our self-esteem, our security, our ambitions, our personal or sex relations which had been interfered with? (Complete each column within Column 3 going from top to bottom. Starting with the Self-Esteem Column and finishing with the Sexual Ambitions Column. Do nothing on Column 4 until Column 3 is complete.)

Instruction 4 Referring to our list again. Putting out of our minds the wrongs others had done, we resolutely looked for our own mistakes. Where had we been selfish, dishonest, self-seeking and frightened and inconsiderate? (Asking ourselves the above questions we complete each column within Column 4.)

Instruction 5 Reading from left to right we now see the resentment (Column 1), the cause (Column 2), the part of self that had been affected (Column 3), and the exact nature of the defect within us that allowed the resentment to surface and block us off from God's will (Column 4).

	COLUMN 1 I'm resentful at:	COLUMN 2 The cause:	"SELF" COLUMN 3 AFFECTS MY (Which part of self is affected?)										COLUMN 4 What is the exact nature of my wrongs, faults, mistakes, defects, shortcomings:			
			Social Instinct		Security Instinct		Sex Instinct		Ambitions							
			Self-Esteem	Personal Relationships	Material	Emotional	Acceptable Sex Relations	Hidden Sex Relations	Social	Security	Sexual	Selfish	Dishonest	Self-Seeking & Frightened	Inconsiderate
1															
2															
3															
4															
5															
6															
7															
8															

4-A

HOW IT WORKS

1. What are the two schools of thought about sex?

   P 69   L 6-8

2. What do we want to stay away from?

   P 69   L 8-9

3. Does the AA text give sex standards?

   P 69   L 9-10

4. Which group of people has sex problems?

   P 69   L 10

5. What is the big question we are all faced with?

   P 69   L 11

6. Where are we told to list the character defects that cause sex problems?

   P 69   L 12-14

7. Where are we told to list the people we have hurt?

   P 69   L 14-16

8. Must we put this on paper?

   P 69   L 16-17

9. What do we learn to do in the future regarding our sex life?

   P 69   L 18-19

10. Should we set new standards for ourselves and test each relation as it occurs?

    P 69   L 19-20

11. What is the sex test?

    P 69   L 20

HOW IT WORKS

12. How do we develop new sex standards?

    P 69   L 20-21

13. Where do we get our sex powers?

    P 69   L 21-22

14. Should this power be thrown away and wasted?

    P 69   L 23-24

15. After we have set new goals, how do we get there?

    P 69   L 25-26

16. What do we do about the problems we had caused because of our sex conduct?

    P 69   L 26-27

17. When do we not make amends for our conduct?

    P 69   L 27-28

18. Is sex the same as our other problems?

    P 69   L 28-30

19. We had a prayer about our resentments and we had prayer about fear. How do we deal with our sex problems?

    P 69   L 30-31

20. Who must judge our sex lives?

    P 69   L 33

REVIEW OF OUR OWN SEX CONDUCT
INSTRUCTIONS FOR COMPLETION

Instruction 1 We listed all people we harmed. (Complete Column 1 from top to bottom. Do nothing on Columns 2, 3 or 4 until Column 1 is complete.)

Instruction 2 We asked ourselves what we did. (Complete Column 2 from top to bottom. Do nothing on Columns 3 or 4 until Column 2 is complete.)

Instruction 3 Was it our self-esteem, our security, our ambitions, our sex instinct, which caused the harm? (Complete each column within Column 3 going from top to bottom. Starting with the Self-Esteem Column and finishing with the Sexual Ambitions Column. Do nothing on Column 4 until Column 3 is complete.)

Instruction 4 Referring to our list again. Putting out of our minds the wrongs others had done, we resolutely looked for our own mistakes. Where had we been selfish, dishonest, self-seeking and frightened and inconsiderate? (Asking ourselves the above questions we complete each column within Column 4.)

Instruction 5 Reading from left to right we now see the harm (Column 1), what we did (Column 2), the part of self which caused the harm (Column 3), and the exact nature of the defect within us that caused the harm, and block us off from God's will (Column 4).

"SELF"

COLUMN 1	COLUMN 2	COLUMN 3 AFFECTS MY (Which part of self caused the harm?)										COLUMN 4 What is the exact nature of my wrongs, faults, mistakes, defects, shortcomings:			
		Social Instinct		Security Instinct		Sex Instinct		Ambitions							
Who did I harm?	What did I do?	Self-Esteem	Personal Relationships	Material	Emotional	Acceptable Sex Relations	Hidden Sex Relations	Social	Security	Sexual		Selfish	Dishonest	Self-Seeking & Frightened	Inconsiderate
1															
2															
3															
4															
5															
6															
7															
8															

HOW IT WORKS

1. What are we being told for the second time about God?
   P 70   L 1-2

2. Do we rely on other people when it comes to advice on sex?
   P 70   L 2-4

3. If we have troubles with sex, will we drink in every case?
   P 70   L 5-8

4. When people have problems with sex, what must they do to keep from drinking?
   P 70   L 8-11

5. If they are not sorry, what will happen to them?
   P 70   L 11-13

6. How did the first 100 know about this?
   P 70   L 14

7. Where are we told to pray about sex the second time?
   P 70   L 15-18

8. What is another weapon given to help us overcome sex problems?
   P 70   L 18-20

9. When working with others, what happens to us?
   P 70   L 20-22

10. As we began to summarize our inventory, what should we have written down?
    P 70   L 23-25

11. What should we learn from our inventory?
    P 70   L 25-26

12. By analyzing them, what do we see?
    P 70   L 26-30

13. Should we have started our list for step 8?
    P 70   L 30-32

14. Is faith a power greater than ourselves?
    P 70   L 33   P 71   L 1

HOW IT WORKS

1. What do we need to be convinced of?
   P 71   L 1-3

2. What blocks us from God?
   P 71   L 3

3. Where should we be after taking steps 3 and 4?
   P 71   L 3-5

4. Does our first inventory get rid of all our handicaps?
   P 71   L 6-7

WORD DEFINITION
HOW IT WORKS

PAGE 58

RARELY: not often; seldom; infrequently

PATH: way of life, conduct or thought

COMPLETELY: totally, absolutely

SIMPLE: not involved or complicated

PROGRAM: plan of action taken toward a goal

CONSTITUTIONALLY: of or proceeding from the basic structure or nature of a person or thing

INCAPABLE: lacking strength, ability or power

UNFORTUNATES: unsuccessful or unsuitable people

FAULT: responsible; open to blame

GRASP: take hold of; intellectually comprehend

RIGOROUS: rigid, severe, harsh, strict

MANNER: the way in which a thing is done or happens

EARNESTNESS: seriousness, eagerness

NIL: nothing, naught, zero

CUNNING: crafty, tricky

BAFFLING: confusing, bewildering

PAGE 59

AVAIL: advantage, use

ABANDON: giving up

RECOVERY: a return to a normal condition

ADMITTED: acknowledged, confessed; admitted the truth

POWERLESS: lacking strength or power; helpless

BELIEVE: accept as true or real

SANITY: whole or sound of mind

DECISION: a course of action chosen

MORAL: correct and true

INVENTORY: a detailed list of things in one's view or possession

EXACT: accurate and specific

NATURE: the basic or essential characteristics of something

DEFECT: deficiency, fault, flaw

CHARACTER: personality in action

HUMBLY: lacking pride; aware of one's shortcomings

SHORTCOMING: deficiency, flaw, fault

AMENDS: the correction of injuries or mistakes

CONTINUE: go on with a particular action

PRAYER: any act of communication with God

MEDITATION: serious comtemplation or reflection; listening for directions

CONSCIOUS: known or felt by one's innerself

CONTACT: the state of being in communication

PAGE 60

AWAKENING: consciousness or awareness

PRINCIPLE: a basic truth or law

ADHERENCE: faithfulness; sticking to

PERTINENT: very significant or important

SOUGHT: tried to find; searched

VIRTUOUS: righteous, pure

EGOTISTICAL: devoted to one's own interest and advancements

INDIGNANT: angry because of an unjust action

DELUSION: false belief held as a result of self-deception

EGO-CENTRIC: thinking or acting with the view that one's self is the center

UTOPIA: ideal, perfect

PROTESTATIONS: objections, disapproval

SELF-PITY: dwelling on one's sorrows or misfortunes

SELFISHNESS: concern chiefly or only with oneself

SELF-CENTEREDNESS: selfishness

SELF-DELUSION: tricking or lying to oneself

SELF-SEEKING: pursuing only for oneself

PROVOCATION: the act of stirring or inciting to action

DIRECTOR: one who supervises, controls or manages

REBORN: born again; emotionally or spiritually revived or regenerated

BONDAGE: subjected to any force, power of influence

STRENUOUS: very active; energetic

MANIFESTED: shown or demonstrated plainly

RESENTMENT: ill will felt because of a real or imagined wrong

OUR POCKETBOOK: supply of money; financial resources

AMBITIONS: goals

GRUDGE: a deep-seated resentment

SELF-ESTEEM: satisfaction with oneself

SECURITY: freedom from risk or danger; safety

PAGE 66
FUTILITY: uselessness; without purpose

SQUANDER: to spend wastefully or extravagantly

GROUCH: a habitually complaining or irritable person

BRAINSTORM: a sudden, clever, whimsical or foolish idea

PAGE 67
SYMPTOMS: evidence of disease

TOLERANCE: allowing or respecting the beliefs or behavior of others

PATIENCE: an understanding of a trying situation or person

RETALIATION: revenge

CORRODING: slowly weakening

PAGE 68
SELF-RELIANCE: dependence upon one's own capabilities of judgment or resources

SELF-CONFIDENCE: trust in oneself or one's abilities

INFINITE: having no boundaries or limits

FINITE: having limited boundaries

PARADOXICALLY: seemingly contradictory but true

OVERHAULING: repairs

EXTREME: excessive degree

ABSURD: ridiculous, unreasonable

PRECREATION: bringing forth; reproduce (offspring)

PAGE 69
SIGNIFICANCE: importance

FLAVOR: something that adds to or enhances

FARE: activities

ARBITER: one chosen or appointed to judge or decide a disputed issue

SELFISH: concerned chiefly or only with oneself

DISHONEST: lacking truth

INCONSIDERATE: careless of the rights or feelings of others; thoughtless

AROUSE: awaken from sleep; rouse to action

JEALOUSY: envious resentment against a successful rival

SUSPICION: doubt or distrust; a feeling that something is wrong without definite evidence

BITTERNESS: painful resentment

MOLD: form into shape

DESPISED: scorned, condemned

LOATHED: disliked greatly; detested

PAGE 70

FANATICAL: excessive; very intense

LOOSE: free from restraint

HYSTERICAL: very emotional

GUIDANCE: advice, direction, leadership

QUESTIONABLE SITUATION: doubtful activity

IMPERIOUS: domineering; overbearing; commanding

URGE: strong desire to do or say something

HEARTACHE: anguish of mind; sorrow

ANALYZED: examined critically

COMPREHEND: grasp the meaning of mentally; understand

FUTILITY: uselessness; without purpose

FATALITY: deadliness

PAGE 71

GROSSER: glaringly noticeable

HANDICAPS: a disadvantage that makes progress or success more difficult

SWALLOWED: taken in mentally

DIGESTED; absorbed or assimilated mentally

CHUNKS: large amounts

CHAPTER 6
INTO ACTION

1. Why are we working the steps?

   P 72   L 2-4

2. What should we have learned if we have taken steps 3 and 4 in the manner the book suggests?

   P 72   L 4-7

3. What are we about to do with the weak items?

   P 72   L 7-8

4. What will it take to complete the job?

   P 72   L 8

5. Do we do the job from the inside out or the outside in?

   P 72   L 8-11

6. Do we need a reason to take step 5?

   P 72   L 19-22

7. What is the best reason for taking this step?

   P 72   L 22-25

8. Why do newcomers try to avoid step 5, and what are they looking for?

   P 72   L 25-26

9. What happens to alcoholics who do not take step 5?

   P 72   L 26   P 73   L 1

INTO ACTION

1. What did they hang on to?

   P 73   L 5

2. What did they think they had done?

   P 73   L 6-7

3. What do we learn in step 5?

   P 73   L 7-10

4. How much of our life story do we have to tell?

   P 73   L 10

5. Does the alcoholic live two lives?

   P 73   L 11-15

6. What happens to the alcoholic in a blackout?

   P 73   L 16-22

7. Do blackouts cause more drinking?

   P 73   L 22-23

8. Do alcoholics go to psychologists and pay them money to listen to lies?

   P 73   L 24-28

9. If we can't talk to our doctor, whom can we talk to?

   P 73   L 28-30

10. What kind of opinion do medical men have of the alcoholic?

    P 73   L 30-32

11. What must we do to have a good life?

    P 73   L 33   P 74   L 1

INTO ACTION

1. Should we be careful when we choose the person with whom we are going to take step 5?

   P 74   L 1-4

2. Can we use our religious preferences in taking this step?

   P 74   L 4-7

3. For those of us who do not belong to a church, can we still use established religion to help us with step 5?

   P 74   L 7-9

4. If we do not want to use a religious person, what can we do?

   P 74   L 13-15

5. Can we use our doctor?

   P 74   L 15-16

6. Can it be a family member?

   P 74   L 16

7. What must we be careful with in talking to friends and parents?

   P 74   L 16-18

8. What can we not do?

   P 74   L 18-20

9. Can we tell some part to someone else?

   P 74   L 20-21

10. What is the rule for taking step 5?

    P 74   L 21-23

11. What are the reasons for postponing step 5?

    P 74   L 26-end

32 lines on this page.

INTO ACTION

1. Can this be used as an excuse?

   P 75   L 1-2

2. When we pick the person, when do we do step 5?

   P 75   L 3-4

3. What do we carry with us to take step 5?

   P 75   L 4-5

4. How do most people feel about helping us with this step?

   P 75   L 8-9

5. How do you take step 5?

   P 75   L 11-12

6. What happens as the result of this step?

   P 75   L 12-21

7. Can we hope for a new outlook?

   P 75   L 14

8. Are we still uptight?

   P 75   L 14-15

9. What happens to our fear?

   P 75   L 15-16

10. To whom are we getting closer?

    P 75   L 16

11. After the fears leave us, does the spiritual experience start?

    P 75   L 16-18

12. Does the urge to drink sometimes leave at this point?

    P 75   L 18-20

13. Where is our hand after step 5?

    P 75   L 20-21

INTO ACTION

14. Does the spiritual experience begin at step 3 or step 5?
    P 75   L 16-18

15. Can we now take a rest?
    P 75   L 22-23

16. For how long?
    P 75   L 23

17. Is there prayer in step 5?
    P 75   L 24-25

18. How do we check on our work this far?
    P 75   L 25-end

19. What is the purpose of the arch we are building?
    P 75   L 27-30

INTO ACTION

1. After we have started this arch in step 3 and added more stones in steps 1, 4 and 5, do we stop again or do we work on?

   P 76   L 1-2

2. What force within us has to be regenerated to take steps 6 and 7?

   P 76   L 2-3

3. What do we now ask ourselves?

   P 76   L 3-5

4. What is wrong with these things?

   P 76   L 4-5

5. Which ones do we want God to take?

   P 76   L 5

6. If we are not willing, what do we do?

   P 76   L 6-7

7. Where is the step 6 and 7 prayer?

   P 76   L 8-14

8. Do we just turn our drinking problem over to God?

   P 76   L 9-10

9. What do we ask him to do for us?

   P 76   L 10-12

10. What benefit is our improvement to God?

    P 76   L 11-12

11. What else do we ask for here?

    P 76   L 12-13

INTO ACTION

12. When we have completed step 6, we have also completed what?

    P 76   L 14

13. Where and when did we make an amends list?

    P 76   L 17-19

14. Did we take step 4?

    P 76   L 19-20

15. What caused the damage with our fellows?

    P 76   L 22-24

16. When do we get the will to take steps 8 and 9?

    P 76   L 24-25

17. Is there prayer in this step?

    P 76   L 24-25

18. What is our motivation for doing this?

    P 76   L 25-27

19. Should we approach these people on a spiritual basis?

    P 76   L 31-end

INTO ACTION

1. What might happen if we approach people this way?

   P 77   L 1

2. What is the first job?

   P 77   L 1-2

3. Will this be the end of our work?

   P 77   L 2-3

4. What is our real purpose?

   P 77   L 3-4

5. What happens when we go to someone we have hurt and tell him we have gotten religion?

   P 77   L 4-9

6. What else could happen?

   P 77   L 9-11

7. What impresses most, demonstration or spiritual conversation?

   P 77   L 12-14

8. Are we ashamed of God?

   P 77   L 15-16

9. How do we express our convictions?

   P 77   L 16-18

10. What question will come up here?

    P 77   L 18-19

11. When others have hurt us more than we have hurt them, how do we feel about amends?

    P 77   L 19-23

12. What must we do with a person we disliked?

    P 77   L 23-24

INTO ACTION

13. Are amends harder to make to an enemy than a friend?

    P 77   L 24-25

14. Do we get more from amends to our enemies than to our friends?

    P 77   L 25-26

15. What do we do when making amends to an enemy?

    P 77   L 26-28

16. What is it that we never do in making an amend?

    P 77   L 29-30

17. Whose side are we trying to clear?

    P 77   L 32-end

INTO ACTION

1. Are we to discuss the other person's faults?
   P 78 L 2-3

2. What should our manner be to make a success of this step?
   P 78 L 3-4

3. What is the percentage of success in making amends?
   P 78 L 5

4. Do we sometimes have others admit their faults to us?
   P 78 L 6-7

5. What are the results?
   P 78 L 7-8

6. Can amends be a failure?
   P 78 L 8

7. Can we make our enemies our friends?
   P 78 L 9-11

8. Do we sometimes run into trouble making amends?
   P 78 L 11-12

9. If we have done our part in the amend and it is not accepted, how should we feel?
   P 78 L 13

10. Do a few alcoholics owe money?
    P 78 L 14

11. Should the alcoholic face his debts?
    P 78 L 14-15

12. Do we tell people we owe money to about our drinking?
    P 78 L 15-16

INTO ACTION

13. Do they already know about it?
    P 78   L 16-17

14. Do we hide our alcoholism due to fear of financial harm?
    P 78   L 17-19

15. Will our creditors surprise us?
    P 78   L 19-20

16. Do we tell our creditors we are sorry?
    P 78   L 21-22

17. What does drinking do the alcoholic's ability to pay his bills?
    P 78   L 22-23

18. What fear must we lose?
    P 78   L 23-24

19. If we don't what will happen?
    P 78   L 24-25

20. What two examples are given of criminal offense?
    P 78   L 28-33

21. Have we talked about this in step 5?
    P 78   L 29-30

22. Have most of us had the same problem?
    P 78   L 33

INTO ACTION

1. What is another common form of trouble that alcoholics have?

   P 79   L 1-4

2. Are these handled in a different way?

   P 79   L 5-7

3. What principle is involved in them all?

   P 79   L 7-8

4. Why are we taking these steps?

   P 79   L 8

5. Do we pray?

   P 79   L 8-11

6. Are we threatened by our past?

   P 79   L 11-12

7. What must we not do?

   P 79   L 12-13

8. Do we save ourselves from alcoholism at the expense of others?

   P 79   L 14-17

9. What have remarried alcoholics failed to do?

   P 79   L 17-19

10. What did his ex-wife do?

    P 79   L 19-20

11. What was this man doing to improve his life?

    P 79   L 20-22

12. What could he have done?

    P 79   L 22-24

INTO ACTION

13. What would have happened if he had done this?

    P 79   L 25-27

14. What did his sponsor tell him?

    P 79   L 27-29

15. What were the results?

    P 79   L 30-end

INTO ACTION

1. What should we do before we involve other people?
   P 80   L 1-2

2. After we ask others, who else do we ask?
   P 80   L 2-4

3. What kind of step is 9?
   P 80   L 4

4. What is it that we must not do?
   P 80   L 4-5

5. In the story that follows:
   1. Did he borrow from an enemy or a friend? P 80 L 7-8
   2. Were other people involved? P 80 L 15-17
   3. Was his financial life involved? P 80 L 17-18
   4. Did he get the consent of others involved? P 80 L 21-22
   5. Did he ask God? P 80 L 24-25
   6. What were his results? P 80 L 28-31
   7. Do alcoholics have extramarital affairs? P 80 L 33 P 81 L 1

INTO ACTION

1. Is the alcoholic any worse than others in these matters?

   P 81   L 1-3

2. What does drinking do to our sex life at home?

   P 81   L 3-4

3. What do we do to our lives?

   P 81   L 4-5

4. How does the alcoholic react to the wife he has made sick?

   P 81   L 6-7

5. What does he look for?

   P 81   L 7-9

6. Does he find it?

   P 81   L 9-11

7. Is there a girl who always understands?

   P 81   L 11-13

8. How does a man feel who has done this?

   P 81   L 13-14

9. What kind of wives are sometimes involved?

   P 81   L 14-16

10. Even in this case, what has to take place?

    P 81   L 17-18

11. Do we tell our wife?

    P 81   L 19

12. Do we give her details?

    P 81   L 19-25

INTO ACTION

13. If she wants to know more, what do we do?

    P 81   L 24-27

14. Do we admit our faults?

    P 81   L 25-27

15. Is there a limitation in what we can do about the matter?

    P 81   L 27-28

16. Is our new way of life just for us?

    P 81   L 32-33

17. What can the alcoholic and his wife both do?

    P 81   L 33   P 82   L 1

INTO ACTION

1. When we give names of other women, what do we do?
   P 82   L 3-8

2. Is there more prayer in making amends?
   P 82   L 8-9

3. What is the most terrible human emotion?
   P 82   L 10-11

4. Do we all make these amends face to face?
   P 82   L 11-13

5. Even if we have no extramarital problems, where should we work?
   P 82   L 14-15

6. Is staying sober enough?
   P 82   L 15-16

7. Does staying sober keep the home intact?
   P 82   L 17-18

8. Does staying sober make amends to our wife and parents?
   P 82   L 18-20

9. What have they shown toward us while drinking?
   P 82   L 20-22

10. What have they saved us from?
    P 82   L 22-23

11. What is the alcoholic like in the lives of other people around him?
    P 82   L 24-25

12. What destruction does he cause?
    L 82   L 25-28

13. What is wrong with a man who says staying sober is enough?
    P 82   L 28-29

INTO ACTION

1. What lies ahead?

   P 83   L 1

2. Who must lead?

   P 83   L 2

3. Is feeling sorry enough?

   P 83   L 2-3

4. What do we do with our family?

   P 83   L 3-4

5. What are we careful not to do?

   P 83   L 5

6. Do our family members have defects?

   P 83   L 6

7. Who caused their defects?

   P 83   L 7

8. Do we pray?

   P 83   L 8-9

9. How often do we pray?

   P 83   L 8

10. What do we ask for?

    P 83   L 9-10

11. Is a spiritual life a theory?

    P 83   L 11

12. How do we get a spiritual life?

    P 83   L 11

INTO ACTION

13. Do we try to influence our family in spiritual matters?
    P 83   L 12-14   *"Unless one's family expresses a desire to live upon spiritual principles."*

14. Should we even talk to them about spiritual matters?
    P 83   L 14-15

15. Will they change?
    P 83   L 15

16. Do our actions speak louder than words?
    P 83   L 15-16

17. What has our drinking done to our family?
    P 83   L 17-18

18. Can we set right all wrongs?
    P 83   L 19

19. Do we worry about them? What do we do?
    P 83   L 20-21

20. What about people who can't be seen?
    P 83   L 22-23

21. Are delays acceptable?
    P 83   L 24-25

22. Do we crawl before people we have harmed?
    P 83   L 26-28

23. How must we work the first nine steps to get the promised results?   *painstakingly*
    P 83   L 29

24. How far in our progress have we come when we have completed the first nine steps?
    P 83   L 30-31

INTO ACTION

25. When will we be amazed?

    P 83   L 30-31

26. What kind of freedom and happiness will we know?

    P 83   L 31-32

27. Do we still run from our past?

    P 83   L 32-33

28. Will we understand serenity and peace?

    P 83   L 33   P 84   L 1

INTO ACTION

1. What is the next thing we see?
   P 84   L 1-3

2. Do we get out of self-pity? 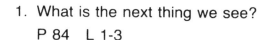 *It will disappear.*
   P 84   L 3-4

3. Do we turn to our fellows?
   P 84   L 4-6

4. Have we had a psychic change?
   P 84   L 6-7

5. What happens to our fears of people and economic insecurity?
   P 84   L 7-8

6. Has our mind improved?
   P 84   L 8-10

7. What is God doing for us?
   P 84   L 10-11

8. Are these too much to expect after working nine simple steps of this 12-step program?
   P 84   L 12

9. Did the first 100 people get this result?
   P 84   L 13

10. Did some of them have a spiritual experience?
    P 84   L 13

11. Did some of them have a spiritual awakening?
    P 84   L 14

INTO ACTION

12. Do these steps only work sometimes?

    P 84   L 14

13. What do we do to get this result?

    P 84   L 14-15

14. Which step are we on at this point?

    P 84   L 16

15. What is the purpose of this step?

    P 84   L 17-18

16. What do we do after completing the nine-step "cleaning up" of the past?

    P 84   L 18-20

17. What spiritual growth have the first nine steps given us?

    P 84   L 20-21

18. Can we stay at this point?

    P 84   L 21-22

19. In what two areas of our lives are we to grow?

    P 84   L 21-22

20. How long must we work at this?

    P 84   L 23

21. Do we continue to work step 4 everyday in our lives?

    P 84   L 23-24

22. When things crop up in life everyday, do we work steps 6 and 7?

    P 84   L 24-25

23. Do we have to use step 5 each day?

    P 84   L 26

INTO ACTION

24. What is our new code?

    P 84   L 29

25. Are we still fighting not to drink?

    P 84   L 30-31

26. In step 2 we came to believe that a power greater than ourselves could restore us to sanity. Is there any growth in our sanity at this point?

    P 84   L 31-32

27. Will liquor be on our minds?

    P 84   L 32

28. What will we do if tempted by alcohol?

    P 84   L 32-end

INTO ACTION

1. What is our new reaction to alcohol?
   P 85 L 1

2. Have we been made whole?
   P 85 L 1

3. What do we find?
   P 85 L 1-2

4. What did this new attitude toward alcohol cost us?
   P 85 L 2-4

5. What could bring about this kind of change in alcoholics?
   P 85 L 4-5

6. How do we feel toward the problem of drinking?
   P 85 L 6-8

7. Have we quit drinking?
   P 85 L 8

8. What happened to the problem?
   P 85 L 8-9

9. What do we have to keep fit to have these promises fulfilled?
   P 85 L 11-12

10. Feeling so much better at this point, what do most alcoholics try to do in this part of recovery?
    P 85 L 13-14

11. What will come if we stop?
    P 85 L 14-15

12. Are we cured?
    P 85 L 15-16

13. Instead of a cure, what do we have?
    P 85 L 16

INTO ACTION

14. What is our sobriety based on?
    P 85   L 17-18

15. How often must we work step 11 to keep spiritually fit?
    P 85   L 18

16. Do we just use God in our spiritual activities?
    P 85   L 19

17. How do we do this?
    P 85   L 19-20

18. What is our 11-step program?
    P 85   L 19-20

19. Do we do this once a day?
    P 85   L 21

20. Can we use our will power properly?
    P 85   L 22-23

21. If we have taken the first 10 steps, what should we sense already?
    P 85   L 26-28

22. What else have we gained as the result of the 10 steps?
    P 85   L 28-29

23. We are born with five senses. What do we develop now?
    P 85   L 29-30

24. What must we do to perfect this gift?
    P 85   L 30-31

25. What does step 11 suggest?
    P 85   L 32

26. What are we warned not to do about prayer?
    P 85   L 32-33

27. What men make use of prayer?
    P 85   L 33   P 86   L 1

INTO ACTION

1. What two things are needed to make prayer work?

   P 86   L 1-2

2. Did the first 100 want to take on the task of directing us in prayer?

   P 86   L 2-3

3. What did they give us to help us develop a spiritual life?

   P 86   L 3-4

4. When is the first suggestion to be used?

   P 86   L 5-6

5. Each night in our review, do we ask if we took step 7 today?

   P 86   L 6-7

6. In our review, do we ask about step 9?

   P 86   L 7

7. In our review each night, do we check out step 5?

   P 86   L 7-9

8. What must we be careful not to do?

   P 86   L 13-16

9. After our review, what do we do?

   P 86   L 16-18

10. When do we use our second suggestion?

    P 86   L 19

11. How far should we think ahead?

    P 86   L 19-20

12. What do we first look at each day?

    P 86   L 20

INTO ACTION

13. Before working our plan, what do we ask God to direct?
    P 86   L 20-21

14. What is the thing we must avoid each day?
    P 86   L 22-23

15. When self is removed, do our minds get better?
    P 86   L 23-25

16. Does the alcoholic have brains?
    P 86   L 25

17. Can the alcoholic ever use his brains better?
    P 86   L 25-26

18. What blocks us from a good thought-life?
    P 86   L 27

19. What do we do about indecision?
    P 86   L 28

20. Do we use prayer here?
    P 86   L 30-31

21. After prayer, what do we do?
    P 86   L 31

22. What is it we must not do?
    P 86   L 31-32

23. After working these suggestions, is there still indecision?
    P 86   L 32-end

INTO ACTION

1. What happens after we work the suggestions for awhile?
   P 87   L 1-2

2. Can new people in the program use step 11 effectively?
   P 87   L 3-5

3. Do we sometimes have trouble trying to understand God's will in our lives?
   P 87   L 4-5

4. Will it cost us?
   P 87   L 5-7

5. Does practice of step 11 enable us to improve?
   P 87   L 7-8

6. After we practice step 11 for a time, what will happen?
   P 87   L 9

7. How do we conclude our meditation?
   P 87   L 10-11

8. What prevents us from reentering into indecision again that day?
   P 87   L 11-13

9. What must we be free of each day?
   P 87   L 13-14

10. Do we tell God what we want?
    P 87   L 14-15

11. Under what condition can we ask God to help us?
    P 87   L 15-16

12. Should we pray asking God to help us with our will?
    P 87   L 16-17

INTO ACTION

13. Why should we not ask God to help us have our way?
    P 87   L 17-19

14. Can we involve our family in our prayer and meditation?
    P 87   L 20-21

15. Does the alcoholic still practice his religious devotion?
    P 87   L 21-23

16. Can an alcoholic who is not a church member use religious prayer?
    P 87   L 23-26

17. What else is helpful to the alcoholic in his meditation?
    P 87   L 26-27

18. Can the alcoholic use counseling by religious leaders in his personal program?
    P 87   L 27-28

19. What must we be quick to see?
    P 87   L 28-30

20. Where is the fifth suggestion used?
    P 87   L 31

21. What does the alcoholic do when agitated?
    P 87   L 31

22. When agitated, what do we pray for?
    P 87   L 32

23. What does the alcoholic need to be constantly reminded of all through each day?
    P 87   L 33   P 88   L 1

INTO ACTION

1. How do we do this?

   P 88   L 1-2

2. What is the result of working step 11?

   P 88   L 2-7

3. Can the alcoholic do more living each day after completing the 11th step?

   P 88   L 4-6

4. Does this level go up?

   P 88   L 5

5. Why?

   P 88   L 5-7

6. Do these steps really work?

   P 88   L 8

WORD DEFINITION
INTO ACTION

PAGE 72

ATTITUDE: mental position or state of mind

CREATOR: God

OBSTACLES: things that stand in the way of progress toward a goal

ADMITTED: confessed to; acknowledged

ASCERTAINED: learned with certainty; found

EXACT: accurate and specific

NATURE: the basic or essential characteristics of something

DEFECTS: deficiencies, faults, flaws

APPRAISAL: finding the value of

INSUFFICIENT: inadequate; not good enough

RECONCILED: made friendly again; settled

VITAL: of first importance; essential

HUMBLING: lowered in pride, importance or dignity; made meek

EGOISM: valuing everything only in reference to one's personal interest

REPUTATION: overall quality or character as seen or judged by others

PAGE 73

EPISODES: incidents, events

VAGUELY: not clearly

PSYCHOLOGISTS: those trained in psychology (the science of mind and behavior

SYMPATHTIC: feeling compassion

PAGE 74

INTIMATE: very personal or private

CONFIDENTIAL: secret

DENOMINATION: body, organization

ESTABLISHED RELIGION: denominations that have existed for a long time

ENCOUNTER: come upon; meet unexpectedly

SUITABLE: appropriate, fitting, becoming

PAGE 75

ILLUMINATING: throwing light on; revealing

SPIRITUAL EXPERIENCE: sudden awareness of a higher power or God

BROAD HIGHWAY: a wide, open, all-inclusive course or way

SPIRIT OF THE UNIVERSE: God

ARCH: gateway

PAGE 76

OBJECTIONABLE: displeasing, offensive

BIDDING: work

DRASTIC: especially severe; extreme

SELF-APPRAISAL: the act of determining the value of self

ACCUMULATED: collected or gathered; increased in quantity, number or amount

ACQUAINTANCE: a person one knows

FRIENDS: those attached to others by affection or esteem

REASSURED: restored to confidence

PAGE 77

MAXIMUM: the greatest or most

FANATICS: people with excessive enthusiasm and intense uncritical devotion

BORES: dull or monotonous people

PAGE 78

FRANK: free and forthright in expressing one's feelings and opinions; outspoken

GRATIFIED: pleased or satisfied

FEUDS: prolonged quarrels

CRIMINAL: forbidden by law

OFFENSE: wrongdoing, infraction, misdeed

PAGE 79

INDIGNANT: anger caused by an unjust act

REPARATIONS: repairing or restoring; making amends for wrong

INNUMERABLE: too many to be numbered; countless

FURIOUS: extremely angry

PAGE 80

DRASTIC: especially severe; extreme

IMPLICATE: involve

CONSENT: approval, agreement

SHRINK: to be shy or reluctant to do something

DISCREDITING: hurting someone's reputation

DISGRACE: humiliate

EXONERATING: clearing from accusation or blame

SLANDER: a false statement that damages another's reputation

RUINOUS: destructive

PAGE 81

FUNDAMENTALLY: basically, primarily

UNCOMMUNICATIVE: not inclined to talk; reserved

REMORSEFUL: feeling distress arising from a sense of guilt for past wrongs

VENT: express, release

EMOTION: a feeling

JEALOUSY: envious resentment against a successful rival

AFFECTIONS: fond attachments

UPROOTED: removed completely

TURMOIL: a state of commotion or disturbance

RECONSTRUCTION: rebuilding; making over

ANALYZE: examine critically

DEFECTS: deficiencies, faults, flaws

SKEPTIC: one who questions the validity or authenticity of something

VALID: sound, just or well-founded

POSTPONEMENT: putting off to a later time; delay

SENSIBLE: reasonable, wise

TACTFUL: knowing what to say or do to avoid offending someone

CONSIDERATE: taking into account in view of another's circumstances

SERVILE: behaving like a slave or an inferior

SCRAPING: bowing low

CRAWL: approach in a slave-like manner

PHASE: stage, part

AMAZED: surprised, astonished

FREEDOM: liberty; absence of restriction

HAPPINESS: a state of well-being; contentment; joy

SERENITY: total calmness; tranquility

PEACE: quiet; harmony in personal relations

EXPERIENCE: knowledge or skill gained by actually doing or feeling certain things

USELESSNESS: not valuable or productive

SELF-PITY: dwelling on one's sorrows or misfortunes

SELF-SEEKING: pursuing only for oneself

ATTITUDE: a mental position or state of mind

OUTLOOK: point of view

FEAR: alarm, dread, panic

ECONOMIC: relating to monetary matters

INSECURITY: uncertainty, instability

INTUITIVELY: knowing immediately without conscious reasoning

BAFFLE: confuse or bewilder

EXTRAVAGANT: beyond reason; excessive

FULFILLED: put into effect; realized

MATERIALIZE: come into existence; become fact

SELFISHNESS: concerned excessively or exclusively with oneself

DISHONESTY: lies, deceitfulness

RESENTMENT: ill will felt because of a real or imagined wrong

IMMEDIATELY: now

LOVE: concern

TOLERANCE: allowing or respecting the beliefs or behavior of others

CODE: a system of principles or rules

RECOIL: to draw back quickly

REACT: act or behave in response to something

SANELY: rationally, sensibly

NORMALLY: naturally

NEUTRALITY: not taking either side; neither for nor against

SAFE: free from harm or risk

COCKY: boldly free and forward; conceited

LAURELS: honor (good name); recognition

SUBTLE: difficult to understand; crafty

FOE: enemy, adversary

CURED: restored to health, soundness or normality

MAINTENANCE: upkeep

STRENGTH: power

INSPIRATION: divine influence

DIRECTION: guidance, supervision

VITAL: of first importance

PRAYER: any act of communication with God

MEDITATION: serious contemplation or reflection; listening for directions

SHY: timid, reluctant

PAGE 86

CONSTANTLY: continually; all the time

VAGUE: not clear

DEFINITE: clear, precise

CONSTRUCTIVE: helpful

REVIEW: to look at or study again

APOLOGY: an admission of error or discourtesy accompanied by an expression of regret

MORBID: not healthful; characterized by gloomy or unwholesome ideas or feelings

DIMINISH: lessen, decrease

INDECISION: wavering between two or more possible courses of action

INTUITIVE: known immediately and without conscious reasoning

RELAX: become less tense or rigid

PAGE 87

HUNCH: a strong intuitive feeling as to how something will turn out

PRESUMPTION: something taken to be true

CONCLUDE: to bring to an end; finish

PRIEST: a person who has the authority to conduct religious rites

MINISTER: one officiating or assisting at a church or religious service

RABBI: master teacher used as a term of address for Jewish religious leaders

AGITATED: stirred up; excited; disturbed

PAGE 88

EXCITEMENT: aroused feelings

ANGER: strong displeasure; rage, wrath, fury

WORRY: fear, anxiety

CHAPTER 7
WORKING WITH OTHERS

1. What is the most effective step to work to keep an alcoholic from drinking?

    P 89   L 1-3   *"Practical experence shows that nothing will so much insure immunity from drinking as intensive work with oth alcoholics.*

2. Will it work when the first 11 steps fail?

    P 89   L 3-4   *"It works when other activities fail".*

3. What is the one thing we do in this step?

    P 89   L 4-5   *Carry this message to other alcohdlis...*

4. Can we be more effective than other people with the sick alcoholic?

    P 89   L 5-6

5. Why is the alcoholic effective with other alcoholics?

    P 89   L 6-7

6. What is it that we can do that others can't?

    P 89   L 6-7

7. What is the nature of the alcoholic's problem?

    P 89   L 7

8. Will the alcoholic find a purpose in life?

    P 89   L 8

9. What does helping the sick alcoholic bring into the life of the recovering alcoholic?

    P 89   L 8-12

10. How often should we do this to get the reward?

    P 89   L 12-14

11. How do we find 12-step work?

    P 89   L 16-18

WORKING WITH OTHERS

12. Can the alcoholic learn to work with others from ministers and doctors?

    P 89   L 16-18

13. Should we try to save drunks?

    P 89   L 18-20

14. How should we work with professionals?

    P 89   L 21-22

15. What makes the alcoholic useful?

    P 89   L 22-24

16. What is the only purpose in 12-step work?

    P 89   L 25-26

WORKING WITH OTHERS

1. When we discover our prospect, what is the first thing we do?

   P 90   L 1-2

2. What do we do if he does not want to stop drinking?

   P 90   L 2-4

3. If we try to persuade the alcoholic, what might happen?

   P 90   L 4

4. What do we tell the family of the alcoholic?

   P 90   L 4-5

5. What must the family of the alcoholic learn?

   P 90   L 5-6

6. When learning the alcoholic really wants to stop drinking, what do we do next?

   P 90   L 7-9

7. Whom do we talk to?

   P 90   L 9

8. What do we need to know about our prospect?

   P 90   L 9-11

9. In what way will we use this information?

   P 90   L 11-13

10. Will the family agree with the way you work with the alcoholic?

    P 90   L 15-16

11. When should we not wait for a binge?

    P 90   L 15-16

12. Do we talk to the alcoholic when he is drunk?

    P 90   L 17

WORKING WITH OTHERS

13. When do we visit the family of a drunk?

    P 90   L 17-18

14. What do we wait for to begin our work?

    P 90   L 18-19

15. After drinking is over, what question is asked by the family?

    P 90   L 19-21

16. What is to happen if the answer is yes?

    P 90   L 22-23

17. How do we describe ourselves to the alcoholic? What do we tell him on the first meeting?

    P 90   L 23-26

18. Do we try to force the new alcoholic?

    P 90   L 27-28

19. Should the family plead with the alcoholic?

    P 90   L 28-29

20. What should the family wait for if the man does not respond?

    P 90   L 30-31

21. Can we leave the Big Book?

    P 90   L 31-32

WORKING WITH OTHERS

1. What will happen if the family becomes overanxious?
   P 91   L 1-2

2. Should the family tell your story to the alcoholic?
   P 91   L 3

3. Is the family a good way to approach the alcoholic?
   P 91   L 4-5

4. What is a better way than the family to approach the alcoholic?
   P 91   L 5-6

5. What should we do if the alcoholic needs hospitalization?
   P 91   L 6-7

6. Can we force hospitalization on him?
   P 91   L 7

7. Who can persuade him to go to a hospital?
   P 91   L 8-9

8. When our man is feeling better, who should set up the meeting?
   P 91   L 10-11

9. Do we bring up the family in our first meeting?
   P 91   L 11-12

10. What do we want the alcoholic free of when we talk to him?
    P 91   L 12-14

11. What do we want the family of the alcoholic to avoid?
    P 91   L 14-15

12. Do we let him get to feeling bad before we talk to him?
    P 91   L 15-16

WORKING WITH OTHERS

13. What does depression do to the sick alcoholic?
P 91   L 16-17

14. Is the doctor who helped get involved in our first talk?
P 91   L 18

15. How do we start?
P 91   L 18-19

16. After awhile, what do we turn to?
P 91   L 19-20

17. What do we tell the new alcoholic?
P 91   L 20-22

18. Do we try to get him to talk?
P 91   L 22-23

19. What is the purpose of his talking?
P 91   L 23-24

20. If he does not want to talk, what do we do?
P 91   L 24-26

21. Should we at this point tell the alcoholic about the 12 steps and the Big Book?
P 91   L 26-27

22. Do we still try to get the message of our first step across?
P 91   L 27-28

23. What do we try to get him to talk about?
P 91   L 30-31

24. When should we say that we are alcoholics?
P 91   L 32-end

WORKING WITH OTHERS

1. How do we describe our condition just before coming to AA?

   P 92   L 1

2. What is the first thing we learned?

   P 92   L 1-2

3. Do we tell how will power failed us?

   P 92   L 2-3

4. Which part of the illness do we discuss first, the mind or the body?

   P 92   L 3-4

5. What chapter is used to show the mental obsession?

   P 92   L 4-8

6. What do we dwell on next?

   P 92   L 9-10

7. Do we show him why will power has not worked for him?

   P 92   L 10-13

8. Can we now talk about the AA book?

   P 92   L 13-15

9. Do we brand him as an alcoholic or is he to make the diagnosis?

   P 92   L 15-16

10. What do we do if he still thinks he can control his drinking?

    P 92   L 16-18

11. What main point do we still try to drive home to the sick alcoholic?

    P 92   L 21-23

WORKING WITH OTHERS

12. What do we want the alcoholic to look at?

    P 92   L 23-24

13. Do sick alcoholics know they are alcoholics?

    P 92   L 24-25

14. Why do doctors not tell alcoholics they are alcoholics?

    P 92   L 26-27

15. Why can we talk to him about his alcoholism? What is it that we have that the doctor does not have?

    P 92   L 28-29

16. What should the sick alcoholic begin to do at this point?

    P 92   L 29-31

17. Does the sick alcoholic become curious about the first steps?

    P 92   L 33   P 93   L 2

WORKING WITH OTHERS

1. What do we let him ask?

   P 93   L 2-3

2. When he does finally ask, what do we tell him?

   P 93   L 3-4

3. Do we try to avoid discussing spirituality for fear of running him off?

   P 93   L 4

4. What is to be made clear to the sick alcoholic regarding his conception of God?

   P 93   L 4-8

5. What is the main thing he must do?

   P 93   L 8-10

6. What kind of language is best in dealing with spiritual matters?

   P 93   L 11-12

7. What causes religious prejudice?

   P 93   L 13-15

8. Should we force our spiritual convictions on another?

   P 93   L 15-17

9. Are some active alcoholics church members?

   P 93   L 18-19

10. Do some active alcoholics have a more religious background than people who are sober?

    P 93   L 19-20

11. If the sick alcoholic has more religion than the sober alcoholic, what might he wonder about the conversation?

    P 93   L 20-21

WORKING WITH OTHERS

12. What will the new man be curious about?

    P 93   L 20-23

13. Is faith alone sufficient?

    P 93   L 24-25

14. What makes faith vital?

    P 93   L 25-26

15. Do we teach religion?

    P 93   L 26-28

16. If an alcoholic is getting drunk, what is wrong with his religion?

    P 93   L 30-31

17. What will our story help the new man see?

    P 93   L 31-33

18. Do we represent any faith?

    P 93   L 33   P 94   L 1

WORKING WITH OTHERS

1. Are the principles of the AA program new principles for men to live by?

   P 94   L 1-3

2. What do we outline for the new man at this point?

   P 94   L 4-7

3. Why are we helping the new man?

   P 94   L 7-10

4. Is the new man obligated to us?

   P 94   L 10-11

5. What is the new man told to do when he recovers?

   P 94   L 11-13

6. Do we pressure the new man?

   P 94   L 15-17

7. Why are we not offended if the new man quits?

   P 94   L 16-18

8. What is one good thing we have accomplished?

   P 94   L 19-24

9. Does the new man like step 5?

   P 94   L 25-28

10. Do we talk about our not liking step 5?

    P 94   L 28-29

11. Why do we tell him we took step 5?

    P 94   L 29-31

12. Do we invite him to an AA meeting?

    P 94   L 31-32

13. Do we try to sell him a Big Book?

    P 94   L 32-end

WORKING WITH OTHERS

1. Do we wear out our welcome?
   P 95   L 1-2

2. Do we give new alcoholics a chance to think?
   P 95   L 2-3

3. What excuse is given if the new man has trouble?
   P 95   L 4-8

4. What is it we never do with a new man?
   P 95   L 10-12

5. What do we let the new man inspect?
   P 95   L 11-12

6. What do we offer the new man?
   P 95   L 13-14

7. What do we tell him we will do?
   P 95   L 14-15

8. If the new man wants money, what do we do?
   P 95   L 16-20

9. Should the new man read the book before he decides on the program?
   P 95   L 21-24

10. Where must the desire to find God come from?
    P 95   L 24-25

11. If he wants to try his way, what do we do?
    P 95   L 27-29

WORKING WITH OTHERS

12. If he wants to follow his religion, what do we do?

    P 95   L 27-29

13. Do we have a monopoly on God?

    P 95   L 29-30

14. What do we have?

    P 95   L 30-31

15. What is one thing alcoholics have in common?

    P 95   L 31-end

WORKING WITH OTHERS

1. What do we do when the prospect does not respond?

   P 96   L 1-3

2. What are we doing when we chase the alcoholic who does not want help?

   P 96   L 4-6

3. What will happen to the new man when we leave him alone?

   P 96   L 6-8

4. Can we hurt others by trying to be too helpful?

   P 96   L 8-10

5. Do we sometimes fail on 12-step work?

   P 96   L 10-11

6. What did the man do when he seemed to fail at 12-step work?

   P 96   L 11-14

7. On the second trip to the new man, what has he accomplished?

   P 96   L 15-18

8. What can we give him?

   P 96   L 18-19

9. Do we help him with step 3?

   P 96   L 19-20

10. Do we offer to do step 5?

    P 96   L 21-22

11. Does he have to use us for step 5?

    P 96   L 21-22

WORKING WITH OTHERS

12. Do we help in matters regarding money?

    P 96   L 23-25

13. Do we deprive our family?

    P 96   L 25-26

14. What must we be certain of before we take an alcoholic into our home?

    P 96   L 28-29

15. What happens if we help an alcoholic with money and shelter?

    P 96   L 29   P 97   L 2

32 lines on this page.

WORKING WITH OTHERS

1. Can we avoid 12-step work?
   P 97   L 3

2. What is the foundation of our recovery?
   P 97   L 4-5

3. Are we to be just do-gooders?
   P 97   L 5-6

4. If we are working with alcoholics, how far do we have to go?
   P 97   L 6-7

5. How often may we have to do this?
   P 97   L 7

6. What are some of the problems we may face in 12-step work?
   P 97   L 7-21

7. Do we let an alcoholic stay in our home for a long time?
   P 97   L 22-23

8. What does this do to the alcoholic and our family?
   P 97   L 23-24

9. If the alcoholic does not respond, do we neglect his family?
   P 97   L 25-27

10. What do we offer the family?
    P 97   L 27-28

11. How can the family help the alcoholic?
    P 97   L 28-30

12. What changes can this program bring about in the family?
    P 97   L 30-32

13. Does the man who really wants to recover need charity?
    P 97   L 33   P 98   L 2

WORKING WITH OTHERS

1. What is the matter with those who want money and shelter before sobriety?

   P 98   L 2-4

2. Do we help those who need this help in recovery?

   P 98   L 4-7

3. Is it just giving?

   P 98   L 8-9

4. What difference does giving make?

   P 98   L 9-10

5. What happens when we provide too much service for the alcoholic?

   P 98   L 10-12

6. For what does the alcoholic clamor?

   P 98   L 12-14

7. What is this kind of talk?

   P 98   L 14-15

8. Does he need his wife back or his job back to get sober?

   P 98   L 15-16

9. What is this man placing before his God?

   P 98   L 17-19

10. Can anyone block us from getting well?

    P 98   L 20-21

11. What is the only condition to get them well?

    P 98   L 21-22

12. What are some of the problems in the alcoholic family?

    P 98   L 23-24

WORKING WITH OTHERS

13. How does the alcoholic treat his family problems?

    P 98   L 24-28

14. Who are the lucky alcoholics?

    P 98   L 28-29

15. Suppose the family is at fault?

    P 98   L 29-31

16. What should he concentrate on?

    P 98   L 31-32

17. What should he avoid like the plague?

    P 98   L 32-end

WORKING WITH OTHERS

1. Why must arguments and fault-finding be avoided?

   P 99   L 1-2

2. How long must this be done before it has an effect?

   P 99   L 2

3. Will the effect be great?

   P 99   L 3

4. What do imcompatible people discover?

   P 99   L 3-5

5. Will the family see and admit their defects?

   P 99   L 5-6

6. What kind of atmosphere comes into the family?

   P 99   L 6-8

7. What makes the family want to go along?

   P 99   L 9-10

8. How can the alcoholic make this thing happen in his family?

   P 99   L 10-14

9. Can we be perfect at all times?

   P 99   L 14-15

10. What do we do to keep away from a drink?

    P 99   L 15-17

11. Should divorced or separated alcoholics go back together right away?

    P 99   L 18-19

12. What should the alcoholic be sure of before he goes back to the other spouse?

    P 99   L 19-20

WORKING WITH OTHERS

13. What should the wife understand?

    P 99   L 20-21

14. Should they go back into the old relationship?

    P 99   L 21-23

15. What is new in the relationship?

    P 99   L 23-24

16. Sometimes should the couple remain apart?

    P 99   L 24-26

17. How does one know when the time is right to go back to one's spouse?

    P 99   L 26-29

18. Does an alcoholic have to have his family back to stay sober?

    P 99   L 30-31

19. Does the wife always come back with recovery?

    P 99   L 31-32

20. What do we remind the prospect?

    P 99   L 33   P 100   L 1

WORKING WITH OTHERS

1. What is the alcoholic's recovery dependent upon?

   P 100   L 1-2

2. Can an alcoholic get well without the family?

   P 100   L 2-3

3. What can happen if the family comes back to soon?

   P 100   L 3-4

4. What do we and the new man do each day in our lives?

   P 110   L 5-6

5. When we look back, what can we see that God has done?

   P 100   L 7-10

6. What will happen if we follow the dictates of our Higher Power?

   P 100   L 10-12

7. What about troubles we are now living with?

   P 100   L 12-13

8. When working with a man and his family, what should we do if there is a quarrel?

   P 100   L 14-18

9. What should we tell the family about the growth of the alcoholic?

   P 100   L 18-22

10. What can we tell the family when they are impatient?

    P 100   L 22-24

11. Can we share our personal experience of our family's recovery?

    P 100   L 25-27

12. What can the alcoholic do when he is spiritually fit?

    P 100   L 31-32

13. What do people say we can't do?

    P 100   L 32   P 101   L 5

WORKING WITH OTHERS

1. Is this necessarily so?
   P 101 L 6

2. Do alcoholics do these things?
   P 101 L 7

3. What is wrong with an alcoholic who cannot do these things?
   P 101 L 7-8

4. What causes the trouble in his mind?
   P 101 L 9

5. Where would a man like this have to go to stay sober?
   P 101 L 10-11

6. Would that keep him sober?
   P 101 L 11-13

7. Have women tried this on their alcoholics?
   P 101 L 13-15

8. Does shielding an alcoholic from alcohol work?
   P 101 L 15-17

9. What happens when an alcoholic tries to shield himself from alcohol?
   P 101 L 18-22

10. What is a rule about drinking places?
    P 101 L 23-25

11. What is the important qualification in this matter?
    P 101 L 24

12. How do we qualify each occasion?
    P 101 L 30 P 102 L 3

WORKING WITH OTHERS

1. What must we check before we go where liquor is served?

   P 102   L 3-4

2. What must our motive be?

   P 102   L 4-5

3. Do we think selfishly?

   P 102   L 5-7

4. If we are shaky, what is better for us to be doing?

   P 102   L 7-8

5. What can happen if things are not right within us?

   P 102   L 9-10

6. How will it be if we are right in our minds?

   P 102   L 10-13

7. Suppose we are with someone who wants to eat at a bar, do we go?

   P 102   L 13-14

8. What do we ask our friends not to do?

   P 102   L 14-16

9. Do people ask the alcoholic to drink?

   P 102   L 17-19

10. What were we doing little by little when we were drinking?

    P 102   L 19-20

11. What are we now trying to do with our social life?

    P 102   L 20-21

12. Can we allow friends to carry us back to withdrawing again?

    P 102   L 21-22

WORKING WITH OTHERS

13. Why must we be able to go any place?

    P 102   L 23-25

14. Should we hesitate about going to a sordid spot?

    P 102   L 25-27

15. What keeps us unharmed when we are on the firing line?

    P 102   L 27-28

16. Why do we keep liquor in our home?

    P 102   L 29-31

17. Do all recovered alcoholics think the same way about keeping liquor in the home?

    P 102   L 32-33

18. How and who makes this decision?

    P 102   L 33   P 103   L 2

WORKING WITH OTHERS

1. Do we take sides on the issues concerning the drinking as an institution?

   P 103   L 3-4

2. Why do we not want to be labeled as reformers?

   P 103   L 5-8

3. How will this affect alcoholics who need our help?

   P 103   L 8-10

4. Can people who hate alcohol have any effect on problem drinkers?

   P 103   L 10-13

5. What hope did the first 100 people have for the AA movement?

   P 103   L 14-16

6. What attitude must we maintain to continue to fulfill this hope?

   P 103   L 16-17

7. Why is this necessary?

   P 103   L 17-18

8. Who caused our problem?

   P 103   L 19-20

9. What have we stopped doing?

   P 103   L 20-21

10. Why did we stop?

    P 103   L 21

WORD DEFINITION
WORKING WITH OTHERS

PRACTICAL: useful; not theoretical

EXPERIENCE: knowledge or skill gained from actually doing certain things

INTENSIVE: concentrated, exhaustive

WORK: physical or mental effort or activity

CONFIDENCE: trust

LONELINESS: without companions; dejected by the awareness of being alone

VANISH: disappear or become invisible

EVANGELIST: zealous preacher

REFORMER: one who urges a person to abandon irresponsible or immoral practices

UNFORTUNATELY: unhappily

PREJUDICE: resentments handed down

HANDICAPPED: at a disadvantage

AROUSE: stir up or excite

COMPETENT: capable, skilled

UNIQUELY: the only one of its kind

COOPERATE: work together; help

CRITICIZE: stress someone's faults

PROSPECT: candidate deemed likely to succeed

BEHAVIOR: how someone acts

RELIGIOUS: the way someone worships God

SPREE: a drinking bout

LUCID: easily understood; clear

FELLOWSHIP: a group of people with the same interests or experiences; mutual sharing

HYSTERICALLY: very emotionally

SPECIFIC: exact

RECEPTIVE: ready or willing to receive favorably

DEPRESSED: in low spirits; dejected

SYMPTOM: evidence of disease

COMMUNICATIVE: talkative

ACCOMPLISHED: achieved

HUMOROUS: funny

ESCAPADE: a carefree or reckless adventure

BAFFLED: confused, bewildered

MENTAL TWIST: inexplainable thinking

INCONSISTENCIES: actions not in agreement or harmony with each other

MALADY: a disease or disorder or the body or mind; ailment

PREVENTS: keeps from happening

FUNCTIONING: operation

SEVERELY AFFLICTED: greatly troubled or injured

DOOMED: condemned to an unhappy destiny

PREDICAMENT: a difficult, perplexing or trying situation

PROTEGE: a person under the care and protection of someone influential who intends to further his career

PAGE 93

AGNOSTIC: a person who believes God is unknown and probably unknowable

ATHEIST: a person who believes there is no God

EMPHATIC: strongly stressed

AROUSING: stirring up

PREJUDICE: resentments handed down

THEOLOGICAL: relating to the study and interpretation of religious faith, practice and experience

PROSPECT: candidate deemed likely to succeed

RELIGIOUS EDUCATION: learning the service and worship of God

VITAL: of first importance

SACRIFICE: give up for the sake of something else

PAGE 94

DENOMINATION: a religious organization uniting in a single body; a number of congregations

CANDIDATE: one who offers himself or is proposed by others for an office, membership, right or honor

PAGE 95

STEER: direct, guide

MORAL: virtuous

HILLTOP: high place

PRODDED: incited, stirred

CONSCIENCE: sense of what is right and wrong

MONOPOLY: exclusive possession

PAGE 96
RESPOND: react favorably

DESPERATE: in extreme need of help

EAGERNESS: strong desire or interest

SITUATION: problem

VOLUME: book

HOMELESS: having no home

FINANCIAL ASSISTANCE: money

DISCRETION: good judgment; caution

INSINCERE: not honest or genuine

PAGE 97
RESPONSIBILITIES: matters that someone is required to take care of

SAMARITAN: one ready and generous in helping those in distress

INNUMBERABLE: too many to be numbered; countless

SANITARIUMS: places that care for the chronically ill

JANGLE: ring loudly

SEDATIVES: drugs that calm or relieve tension

PAGE 98
CHARITY: help for the needy

INCONSISTENT: not uniform

CLAMORS: insists loudly

ARGUMENT: dispute, quarrel

FAULT-FINDING: pointing out blame

PLAGUE: an epidemic disease causing a lot of deaths

PAGE 99
TANGIBLE: capable of being seen

PAGE 100

PERSIST: press on resolutely

PARTICIPATE: take part in

QUARRELS: fights or squabbles

PAGE 101

SHUN: avoid deliberately

SHIELD: protect

LEGITIMATE: what is right or in accordance with standards permitted

WHOOPEE PARTIES: drinking and gaiety

VICARIOUS: imagined by being with others

ATMOSPHERE: a surrounding influence or environment

PAGE 102

APPREHENSION: fear of the future

HESITATE: be reluctant; hold back

PAGE 103

INTOLERANCE: unwillingness to allow or respect the beliefs or behavior of others

BITTERNESS: painful resentment

NOTES

NOTES

NOTES

NOTES

NOTES

Other titles that will interest you......

Recovery Dynamics
Joe McQ

Recovery Dynamics is a comprehensive program of instructions and self help materials developed from the text Alcoholics Anonymous for the Treatment Setting.

The Steps We Took
Joe McQ

This is a book of plain-spoken wisdom for people with addictions and people who love them. The author had been a student of the Twelve Steps for thirty one years, and has lectured in 48 states and most major countries.

Decision Guidebook Steps 1-3
This contains the facts of the First 2 Steps and how to make the decision Step 3.

Action Guidebook Steps 4-9
This book contains all the material and instructions of how to take the action steps including the inventory sheets.

Continued Growth Guidebook Steps 10-12
This book gives the new person all they need to grow for the rest of their life.

For price and order information, please call our Telephone Representative.

✗ Kelly Foundation, Inc.
2801 W. Roosevelt Road
Little Rock, AR 72204
Phone: (501) 663-6553 • Fax: (501) 663-6577 • 1-800-245-6428
www.kellyfdn.com • e-mail at Kellyadm@kellyfdn.com